The Business of Medicine:
The Patient a Revenue Stream,
The Physician a Tool
Your Sixth Psychiatric Consultation
William Yee M.D., J.D
Copyright Applied for Jan. 11th, 2020

I was a medical student in Detroit, Michigan from 1968 to 1972.

I have been practicing medicine in Michigan, Indiana, Kentucky and California without interruption since 1972. I am recently licensed in Texas. Another adventure awaits.

I have watched medicine morph from an office with a shingle, "Dr. Do Good," to, "Corporate Medicine."

In 1968 any doctor could graduate from medical school, have a year of internship and then work in a hospital emergency room or rent an office and start a medical practice.

In 1970 I examined a patient at Sinai Hospital in Detroit. I told the patient I could find no medical illness and that I was confused. The patient explained, "My doctor puts me into the hospital one week a year for a rest and complete examination."

"I belong to the UAW and that is a health benefit."

I worked in an automobile factory from 1965 through the summer of 1970 and was a member of the UAW, the United Auto Workers Union. It never occurred to me to take a week's rest in a hospital for a complete physical examination. Every patient teaches me something.

In 1970 Blue Cross, Blue Shield paid doctor's bills and that was it. That was all going to change.

As a medical student at Detroit General Hospital from 1970 to 1972 I did lumbar punctures, liver biopsies, aspirated pleural effusions, and held retractors during surgery. "See one, do one, teach one," was the environment at Detroit General Hospital.

In fact, I did my first spinal tap without seeing one and without supervision. I was told to do it. I obtained the kit and read the instructions.

Relying on what I learned in my anatomy class in the first year, I obtained the spinal fluid without complications. It is a simple procedure if there are no complications.

I was lucky. There were no complications.

Around 1970 I did a rotation in Obstetrics and Gynecology at Hutzel Hospital which was also known as Women's Hospital. I assisted in the delivery of a baby.

The attending became irritated because I wasn't pulling hard enough on the forceps. I was afraid of pulling the head off the baby. He bullied me into pulling harder. I am easily bullied.

I was lucky, the baby didn't even have a bruise from the forceps. The mother and baby were both healthy and without injury. I resolved not to deliver any more babies. It was too stressful for me.

I marvel at the thought that the mother had more babies. The mother had more intestinal fortitude than I did. I confess. I do not like stress and avoid it at every opportunity.

I was on call one night and went to assist with a delivery. The attending was drunk and did not allow me to do more than observe.

The anesthesiologist told the attending that she was going to report him for being drunk.

The doctor responded with invectives and frequent use of the "F" bomb.

He did an episiotomy.

An episiotomy is a surgical cut made at the opening of the vagina during childbirth, for an easier and faster delivery. The episiotomy prevents rupture of tissues during childbirth and injury to the baby from prolonged delivery.

He was taking a long time sewing the patient.

The anesthesiologist became angrier and angrier and told the doctor that he had better not be doing a tubal ligation because the patient had not signed a consent for a tubal ligation.

The doctor responded with more loud cursing.

I told my proctor, the resident in training supervising me, and he said that the hospital had been protecting that doctor for years and there had been prior complaints about his drinking. The Business of Medicine includes the Politics of Medicine, another book later.

I talked to one of the staff doctors and he told

me that the anesthesiology department had been changed from private practice to salaried anesthesiologists. He said he did not like it. He said that in the past a surgeon would select an anesthesiologist to assist with the surgery.

He said that now the hospital assigned an anesthesiologist for the surgery. He added that sometimes the anesthesiologist would be managing two surgeries simultaneously and would go back and forth between the surgical rooms during the surgical procedures. He did not like that part of the change either.

The hospital is in the business of medicine. The hospital has a huge impact on how doctors practice medicine. Doctors are bullied a lot.

As a medical student I found the Friday Mortality and Morbidity Review in the Department of Surgery the most interesting. All deaths and adverse results were reviewed during this meeting with all the surgeons, residents in training and medical students.

The facts and circumstances were laid out in detail. The treatments were analyzed from start to finish and it was determined if there were any alternative treatments that might have improved the outcome.

This was basically a root cause analysis.
If a root cause was identified the department
discussed an error trapping strategy that
would force a better outcome in the future.

"Error trapping," went into my toolbox.

"Forcing a better outcome," went into my
toolbox.

In 1972 I went to Lafayette Clinic as my first
year of training in psychiatry.

Lafayette Clinic was the psychiatric
centerpiece for the Michigan Department of
Mental Health.

It was a psychiatric research hospital. Every
patient had to sign an agreement to participate
in medical research before they could be
admitted to Lafayette Clinic.

Jacques Gottlieb was the director of Detroit's
Lafayette Clinic. I was told that he studied
under Sigmund Freud and was intent on
finding the cure for Schizophrenia. He was able
to obtain huge federal grants for research on
schizophrenia. The reason was that one half of
the nation's hospital beds were occupied by the
severely mentally ill, most of whom were

diagnosed with schizophrenia.

His grants were so huge that he was able to command an annual salary greater than the governor of the state of Michigan.

A cure for schizophrenia was a prize greater than anything that the governor of the state of Michigan could offer.

For the first few weeks patients were examined intensively by psychiatrists, psychologists, social workers, and activity therapists for a comprehensive evaluation. This included physical and laboratory examinations.

Medications were not started until after the evaluation was completed. The arguments among the professors were occasionally quite heated. The Politics of Medicine, another book.

In 1972 the state of Michigan reduced funding for Lafayette Clinic. The insurance companies stopped paying for billing submitted by medical students.

The psychiatric staff were now required to provide a minimum of twenty hours of billing per week. This was culture shock and there was dismay among the clinical staff.

Insurance companies were taking control of the practice of medicine.

Since this was my first year this was my normal. When I was an intern, I did not receive my paycheck unless all my history and physical examinations had been completed for the week.

I was used to providing sixty hours of billing per week and twenty hours was a cake walk. C'est la vie?

I met another resident in training who had a diagnostic problem.

I said, "just do a lumbar puncture."

He responded. "I have never done a lumbar puncture."

I was shocked. I had been doing lumber punctures as a medical student at Detroit General Hospital. It never occurred to me that you could get through medical school and internship without doing a lumbar puncture.

There was a huge variance among psychiatric residents in prior training and experience. All medical students and interns in medicine during the first year after graduating from medical school did not receive the same training. Medical students at Detroit General Hospital did a great deal of medical care and functioned as doctors as juniors and seniors

I completed my first year after medical school at Lafayette Clinic in a straight Psychiatric Internship and became licensed to practice medicine. My first year as a psychiatric resident was also my internship. This was an inducement to enter into residency in psychiatry. Psychiatry was not a popular residency program because it promised a low income after completion of training.

Lafayette Clinic did not allow moonlighting by its residents in training.

In 1973 I transferred to Northville State Hospital so that I could start moonlighting in the Detroit General Hospital Emergency Room.

Dr. Krome ran the Detroit Hospital Emergency Room in 1972 and started a residency training program for Emergency Medicine, one of the first.

I only had a year of internship and was working as an emergency room physician.

Most of the emergency room physicians at that time had no residency training in emergency room medicine.

Dr. Krome told me that I had to write the lab slips and draw the blood samples.

He explained that the insurance companies would not pay if the nurse wrote the lab slips and drew the blood. I had no prior experience so that was my normal. However, it shows how insurance companies can control and dictate medical practice.

One night I saw one hundred patients between 9:00 pm and 7:00 am in the Detroit General Hospital Emergency Room. That was ten patients an hour, six minutes per patient. That was my normal as I had no prior experience.

I did mouth to mouth CPR and drunk in the Detroit Hospital Emergency room. A resident and training and some medical students went to get the CPR mask.

It turned out the drunk was just breathing shallowly so I stopped. When the resident and students returned and started CPR I watched. When they got it right, I told them it wasn't necessary.

They stopped. I thought it was kind of funny.

I was lucky, this was 1973-1974 and before AIDS. I didn't get Hepatitis C or TB.

When I was in training at Northville State Hospital a lady in her nineties aspirated her pureed diet and went into respiratory arrest.

I did mouth to mouth CPR for the second time. It was useless. The pureed diet had clogged her trachea. All I did was push air into her stomach as it could not go to her lungs.

I have done CPR twice. On both occasions it was not effective. On both occasions it was mouth to mouth without protection.

I am lucky, I do not have Hepatitis C or AIDS.

Not everyone is lucky.

While I was at Northville State Hospital, I found out that violent mentally ill patients from all over Michigan were transferred to Northville and released into Detroit.

One of many reasons for Detroit's demise. The Business of Medicine is imbedded in the culture and politics of the locality.

I read about women being murdered in Board and Care homes in Detroit. These women were being paid five or six hundred dollars a month to provide a room for the patients released from Northville State Hospital.

They might house three or four patients and thought they were getting a lot of money.

I may receive letters stating the amount is wrong and they may have been required to provide meals also. It doesn't matter.

I was called to a unit about 11:00 pm. The nurse offered to share her Chinese carry out dinner with me. I told her that my mother was a nurse.

We sat eating and talking. I noticed that it was unusually quiet. I asked the nurse why it was so quiet.

She answered, "at bedtime, everyone receives one hundred milligrams of Mellaril Suspension."

I put that thought into my tool box.

One hundred milligram of Mellaril or Thorazine at bedtime is effective for sleep and a calm psychiatric unit. The "Business of Medicine" includes a quiet and safe night's sleep.

I completed my residency training in 1975. In 1975 the DSM-II dropped homosexuality as a mental illness.

The DSM-II was the second version of the Diagnostic and Statistical Manual of Mental Disorders, originally published by the American Psychiatric Association in 1968.

It was at that time that I realized that the DSM in its various versions was a proprietary system for diagnosing mental illness. I also realized that the DSM-II was based upon politics and a business model and not on pure science.

As a proprietary diagnostic system, the DSM-III was subject to the copyright laws and could not be used unless licensed. The Business of Medicine has many faces.

As homosexuality was no longer a mental illness, insurance companies would no longer pay for the treatment of homosexuality.

There were psychiatrists who specialized in

treating homosexuality as a mental illness in 1975. They were effectively out of business. So many variables can affect your career as a psychiatrist.

After completing my residency training at Northville State Hospital, I applied for a position as a Staff Psychiatrist at Henry Ford Hospital in Detroit. There was only one position.

I was not a chief resident. I didn't think that I had any special qualifications and expected someone else to get the position. I applied anyway.

When Dr. Bresnahan interviewed me for the position he did not inquire about my training in psychoanalysis or psychiatry.

He asked me questions about my work in the Detroit General Hospital Emergency Room.

I told Dr. Bresnahan I used a ten milligram Valium syringe to interrupt seizures.

I explained that I gave it slowly, intravenously, to avoid respiratory arrest and stopped at 5mg when the seizures stopped.

I told him about using intravenous atropine for the treatment of a suicide attempt by malathion poisoning. I told him that the patient had muscle tremors and was foaming at the mouth and after receiving intravenous atropine the patient's muscle tremors stopped and she woke up complaining of a dry mouth.

I told him about seeing one hundred patients in ten hours, doing the history and physicals, writing the lab requests and drawing the blood.

He offered me the position and I took it.

He did not say anything about the other candidates. I did not ask.

I suspect a lot of the graduating residents in Detroit applied for the position. I was lucky. It was the best possible starting position after residency training.

I received the widest possible exposure to psychiatric consultations with the various medical and surgical specialties.

My interest and experience in Emergency Medicine at Detroit General Hospital was what got me the job at Henry Ford Hospital.

Many psychiatric residents had very limited experience in practicing medicine outside of psychiatry.

There were over 800 psychiatric consultations per year with the medical surgical services at Henry Ford Hospital.

I did every third consultation with the Medical Surgical Services in 1975-1976 with Dr. Bresnahan and Dr. Pope doing the rest.

Dr. Bresnahan resigned and I did every other consultation in 1976-1977 with Dr. Pope.

While at Henry Ford Hospital I taught psychiatric residents in training and medical students the art of psychiatry as I knew it.

One of the residents had a family drive a patient from the Henry Ford Hospital Emergency Room to the Detroit General Hospital Emergency Room.

The patient was suicidal and jumped out of the family car on the freeway. After that, patients were always transferred by ambulance.

There was a lot of hostility between the medical staff and administration at Henry Ford

Hospital. Almost all of the staff were salaried. The pay was relatively low for the amount of work being done.

Henry Ford Hospital had a substantial revenue stream taken from the clinical work of the doctors. It was a sweatshop and, "Dr. Burnout," was always an issue there from what I saw.

In any case, the Business of Medicine includes doctors sharing their incomes with hospitals for the privilege of working at hospitals.

The doctors are salaried. It is actually the hospital that decides what the cost of the doctor visit is going to be.

A resident in training at Henry Ford Hospital was dismissed because he was being prosecuted for prescribing controlled substances inappropriately.

Prescribing addicting medication can put you in jail. I put that thought into my radar.

That is another dimension of root cause analysis and error trapping. Learn by the mistakes of others.

An entrepreneur in Flint was sending busloads

of people to Detroit, paying them $100 and a free meal to collect prescriptions for methamphetamines, sleeping pills and tranquilizers.

I had patients coming to me who were receiving methamphetamines in the morning for weight control, valium three times a day for anxiety and a sleeping pill at night.

They could sell the ninety valiums for $450, the thirty methamphetamine pills for $300 and the thirty sleeping pills for $300, a total of $1,050 per month to supplement their monthly government checks.

They were disappointed when I advised them that I did not prescribe addicting medications on a long-term basis.

Diversion of addicting medications into the black market is another face of the Business of Medicine.

I asked for a raise from $42,000 per year to $45,000 per year. I was told, "no."

I asked, "why not? I am generating more than one hundred thousand a year in revenues?"

He answered, "if I gave you $45,000 a year, you would be making more than the acting chairman for the department of psychiatry."

I responded, "I am board-certified, he is not. You have my thirty-day notice."

I then started looking for a job. I was offered $85,000 a year. I was wondering if I would be offered any kind of job and I more than doubled my income. What a shock.

I wondered why anyone would stay at Henry Ford Hospital.

The business of medicine is complicated and confusing to a recently graduated resident in psychiatry.

After I left Henry Ford Hospital, I often returned for the Friday afternoon Grand Rounds.

I was startled when they discussed a suicide that occurred at Henry Ford Hospital. Usually this kind of information is protected by the confidentiality privilege between the doctor and patient.

However, it must have been a matter of public record. There must have been a lawsuit and leaks to the press.

The presentation described a pediatric surgeon who had received an award for being an outstanding doctor for the year. He then asked for a raise and was denied the raise.

He became depressed.

As a medical staff he was not admitted to the F1 ground floor psychiatric unit.

He was admitted to a tenth or eleventh floor private room for treatment of his depression.

He wrote a suicide note and jumped out of the window.

This case was chosen for a Grand Rounds presentation due to the hostility between the medical staff and the administrative staff at Henry Ford Hospital.

It was an opportunity to publicize the sweatshop nature of Henry Ford Hospital.

The "Business of Medicine," has many faces indeed. Henry Ford was opposed to unions and I suppose Henry Ford Hospital was ripe for a doctor's union. I don't think that it happened.

On another visit to Grand Rounds I was confronted with a case from Northville State Hospital.

I don't recall if the case was presented at Grand Rounds or if the case was in fact brought to my attention by the psychiatrist herself.

In any case, it was a matter of public record because it was the subject of both criminal prosecution and civil suit in the courts.

The basic facts are that the psychiatrist had worked her usual 8:00 am to 5:00 pm day. She had examined all three patients. All three patients were on both suicide and homicide precautions.

After 11:00 pm and before 7:00 am there were only two psychiatric technicians on duty for the unit of thirty to forty patients.

The patients were assigned to rooms of four to six beds per room.

During the hours of 11:00 pm and before 7:00 am the two technicians locked themselves in the nursing station because it was not safe to be out on the unit. The state might claim they were safe, but chose to sleep. Point of view?

During the hours of 11:00 pm and before 7:00 am two of the patients on suicide and homicide precautions took a pillow and smothered the third patient on suicide and homicide precautions.

The body was not discovered until the next morning.

The psychiatric technicians were locked in the nurses' station for safety (sleeping?) and not doing their fifteen-minute safety checks. It was too dangerous (sleeping?) to do the safety checks.

The state of Michigan fired the psychiatrist and blamed the death on the psychiatrist.

The two patients were tried and convicted for the murder of the third patient.

The Psychiatrist was later reinstated with back pay. It was determined that she had worked her full eight-hour day, examined both patients, written progress notes and orders as required and could do no more.

The death of the patient was not her fault.

However, she suffered a great deal of stress with damage to her reputation.

She now had record that she had been the subject of a lawsuit that she would have to explain during every job application for the rest of her life.

The "Business of Medicine," in the state hospital system is to control costs.
Staffing at below safe levels saves money.
Another face of the "Business of Medicine."

Working for a state hospital or a state prison can be risky for your life and your professional reputation. Another caution for my radar.

I had worked at Northville State Hospital and had been called to the units many times between 11:00 pm and 7:00 am. I had not noticed that the psych techs had been locking themselves into the nursing station because they came out to greet me.

On one occasion in 1973, about midnight, I was

called to a unit for an emergency.

I got dressed, drove from the on-call night quarters to N or M or whatever building housed the emergency.

When I arrived, I was shown a naked body in the blood-stained snow. The body was already cool.

We brought the body into the building. The eyes were dilated and fixed, a sign of brain death. There was no pulse or respiration.

The psych tech was very distraught.

I asked, "would you like to learn CPR?"

He answered, "yes."

I showed him how to do CPR. He did it very well. It was useless. The patient had no blood to carry oxygen from his lungs to his heart and brain.

The air exchange was good, but there was no blood flowing with the cardiac compressions.

A few months later the Joint Commission surveyed the hospital for accreditation.

Hospitals must be accredited by the Joint Commission or the insurance companies will not pay for psychiatric hospital services.

After the survey, the Joint Commission surveyors interviewed the residents in training in private.

We were asked if there was anything that we knew that needed to be corrected.

I advised the surveyors of the patient wo had stripped himself of clothes and jumped through a small window, and bled to death in the snow from a lacerated femoral artery.

I advised the surveyors that CPR could not make a difference in that patient.

However, this was a large hospital with many patients and many staff. It takes too long for the resident on call to respond to an emergency for CPR to be effective.

I advised the surveyors that all the staff should be trained in CPR, because, sooner or later it would make a difference.

The next month I was assigned to a group to

train all of the employees in CPR. That was 1974. Every hospital I have worked at since then has all the staff trained in CPR.

When AIDS became a medical issue around 1983 many health care practitioners had anxiety about training with CPR because of the risk of transmission of AIDS with CPR.

Everything has a price. The price is not always measured in money. There is risk to life, limb, reputation, and future employment.

The Joint Commission has a large say in how the "Business of Medicine," is conducted. It requires CPR training at accredited health care facilities.

I later joined a multispecialty group in Taylor, Michigan.

The doctors were making money hand over fist, and I was truly amazed. The doctors were investing in Picasso paintings and retirement homes in Hilton Head, South Carolina.

The patients came to me expecting me to prescribe methamphetamine to lose weight, valium for anxiety and sleeping pills for insomnia.

When I explained to them that these medications were only for short term use, they were disappointed.

When I explained to these patients that after prolonged use medications for anxiety, insomnia and pain had rebound insomnia, anxiety and pain worse than what they had before starting the medications, they argued with me.

"Why would my last doctor prescribe these medications if that were true?"

I answered, "you can go to your last doctor and continue these medications. I am not required to prescribe addicting medications."

I spent ninety minutes examining a patient and diagnosed addiction.

I only charged $15 because I knew the patient was going to complain. I was called into the business manager's office to answer for a patient complaint.

I advised the business manager that the patient was a drug addict. I added that I only charged fifteen dollars because I knew the patient was going to complain, and I wanted to make a point of the fact that I was not exploiting the patient in any way.

The business manager was not satisfied.

That is another face of the "Business of Medicine."

I did not fit in and my contract was not renewed at the end of the year.

I was not good at the, "Business of Medicine." My revenue stream was a disappointment.

Integrity in the practice of medicine is the first sacrifice in the Business of Medicine, "making money."

I did not last long with this multispecialty group.

I opened my own office and 100% of my patients came from referral by other doctors.

I made $160,000 a year and after business expenses paid taxes on $112,000 a year from 1978 through 1983.

During that time, I had met other doctors who had encounters with managed care.

Managed care were third parties that controlled services paid for by insurance companies. They were not going to pay for a week in the hospital for a rest and complete physical examination.

I met John Boaz at a party. He was a resident at Lafayette Clinic and graduated AOA from medical school. He was at the top of his class and extremely intelligent. He was unusually happy, and I asked him what good fortune had elevated him so. He answered, "I just received my annual performance bonus, and it was larger than my annual salary." I wanted to know how he did it. Maybe I could cash in too.

"I work for a managed care company. When patients are in the ER, I give them an appointment instead of admitting them."

I met John at another party and he seemed rather glum, "what happened, John, you were so happy at the last party?"

"I gave a patient an appointment instead of admitting him to the psychiatric hospital He went home and committed suicide and the managed care company fired me."

I later learned that the managed care company failed and was purchased by another managed care company.

The learning curve for managed care companies included a lot of collateral damage.

The Business of Medicine is based upon cash flow and profit margin and the learning curve is long and difficult for MBA's with little understanding of the complexities of medicine.

I suppose the reader should read about the Ford Pinto and "Fatalities Associated with Crash Induced Fuel Leakage and Fires for submission to the NHTSA." The decision not to reduce the risk of fires in a crash was carefully considered. Ford Motor Company decided not to invest $11 per car at a cost of $137 million because the cost of deaths and serious injuries would only amount to $49.5 million.

When this was presented to the jury in Grimshaw v. Ford Motor Co., in February 1978, the jury awarded the victim $125 million in punitive damages to discourage corporate indifference to human suffering and death.

As a physician I have sworn the Hippocratic Oath, first, to do no harm. This is not the attitude of attorneys, businessmen or politicians, who, like the Hatfield's and McCoy's, can be vicious on the playing field.

After I left Henry Ford Hospital, I was reading in the papers about Charfoos and Charfoos receiving ten million, dollar settlements for cases coming out of Hudsel Hospital/Women's Hospital in Detroit.

I often wondered if this was because the surgeons were no longer able to select from private practice anesthesiologists and were forced to use the salaried anesthesiologists employed by the hospital.

I read a case where the Hudsel Hospital/Women's Hospital decided not to pay the $10,000,000 settlement and the jury awarded $32,000,000. I often wondered if the issues were similar to the Ford Pinto. Perhaps the reader will send me a note with the facts?

My first encounter with managed care resulted from a consultation in the intensive care unit of Outer Drive Hospital, in Down River Detroit.

The patient had taken an overdose of Elavil As a suicide attempt.

At that time Elavil was known to be very toxic and lethal as an overdose. I had read an anecdotal report of a patient dying after ingesting 1500mg of Elavil. The therapeutic dose of Elavil is 300mg at bedtime. 1500mg is only a five-day supply of Elavil.

I determined that the patient was suicidal and needed to be admitted to a psychiatric hospital for treatment until she was stable and no longer suicidal. I ordered an ambulance transfer to a psychiatric hospital.

I received my very first call from a managed care company. They asked me to discharge the patient and tell the patient to drive to the psychiatric hospital. I advised the managed care company that the patient was suicidal, and that the ambulance transfer was necessary for the patient's safety.

I submitted a bill for $150 dollars or thereabouts for my time and trouble.

I received a, "Dear John," letter from the

managed care company. The letter stated that my bill would not be paid. The reason was that the patient was being treated for an overdose of Elavil, and that was substance abuse, and treatment for substance abuse was not a covered benefit according to the patient's policy.

The patient was treated for depression and a suicide attempt and the managed care company was perpetrating a fraud by reframing the treatment as for substance abuse for the purpose of denying the payment.

However, the time and cost of securing the money was a waste of my time. The managed care company won be default.

Another face of the Business of Medicine.

Insurance companies burden the practicing physician with detailed billing procedures and every error is an opportunity to deny payment. The insurance companies can be very creative in finding "errors," to justify denial of payment.

My referrals came 100% from other physicians. I did all of the consultations to keep their business.

As a result, I did many consultations on patients without insurance and many of the patients with insurance did not pay the deductible or copay.

As a result, when I left private practice in 1984, I left about $250,000 in uncollected billing.

Managed care forced me out of private practice in 1984. All of a sudden all of my patients were assigned to panels of doctors. I was not on any of the panels. I had to close my practice.

I had two patients who offered to pay out of pocket. I told them they should make the insurance company pay for their treatment.

Also, I noticed that when I received checks from Blue Cross/Blue Shield and other insurance companies, the return address was marked, "do not forward, return to sender."

When I left private practice in Michigan and went to Indiana in 1984, I received no forwarded checks from any insurance company.

Another face of the Business of Medicine.

I have been chiseled out of money by just about every means possible over the years. I am not alone.

Many physicians have suffered "Physician Burnout," and abandoned medicine for retirement or alternative employment opportunities. Perhaps, working for the insurance companies?

Before I left my private practice, I was elected Chairman of the Department of Psychiatry at Heritage Hospital in Taylor, Michigan.

I must say, during that period I learned a lot about the Politics of Medicine. It can get quite ugly. That is going to be another book.

A psychiatrist drove from California to Michigan in a red Ferarri. I marveled that a psychiatrist could make enough money to buy a Ferarri. I was driving a Chevrolet Chevette. A Chevette is a subcompact car with a small four-cylinder engine.

Of course, he was hired by the multispecialty group that was making money hands over fist. He probably was investing in Picasso's.

As the Chairman of the Department of Psychiatry I was involved in credentialing him for privileges to practice psychiatry at Heritage Hospital.

Let's call him Dr. Red Ferrari as I do not recall his name, but I recall his car.

Within less than a year his name was in the newspapers.

The facts are alleged in the newspapers that he was treating a surgeon's wife. He burned through the forty or so visits that Blue Cross paid for annually and continued treating the surgeon's wife. It was alleged that he treated the wife and submitted billing under the wife's husband's Blue Cross insurance.

Of course, in order to submit the billing, he had to assign a mental illness to the Surgeon.

Blue Cross sends a notice of billing and diagnosis to the insured. When the surgeon was sent a notice of the treatment by a psychiatrist for a mental illness, he filed a complaint with the insurance company and the police were invited to the party.

Dr. Red Ferrari was charged with crimes and left the state of Michigan. Within a few weeks I received a letter from a mental health facility in the state of Maine asking for references.

I did not know how the prosecution was proceeding. I was afraid that if I said anything negative about Dr. Red Ferrari, he would sue me for libel and slander.

I responded by stating that I did not know Dr. Red Ferrari long enough to say anything positive or negative about him. I was being careful.

Later, I worked in a psychiatric hospital for about seven years. During that time, I was forced to call a doctor working for the insurance company for prior authorization. If the insurance company denied prior authorization the hospital treated the patient without payment.

The call to the insurance doctor is sometimes called a peer to peer review. The insurance doctor asked questions. His job was to ask questions to find a reason to deny payment.

For example, if the patient was not seen every day, there was "no active treatment," and payment for the hospital admission was denied.

If there was no medication change, "there was no active treatment," and additional hospital days were denied for payment.

If the patient was present for longer than four or five days, the care was, "not acute care."

"Chronic care," is not a covered service. Additional days are denied for payment.

The number of days is arbitrary and different from reviewer to reviewer and insurance company to insurance company.

The basis of the denials is largely economic, and the clinical situation is seen differently by the treating psychiatrist and the insurance psychiatrist.

The treating psychiatrist does not want to discharge a suicidal patient home, even if it is past the arbitrary five day, ten day, or fifteen day time period for the "customary length of stay." This time period varies from location to location and from insurance company to insurance company. The duration of stay and the criteria for denial of payment are "trade secrets," that amount to a competitive advantage among the insurance companies.

I kept a patient in a hospital for eight months because he was suicidal. He was released a month later from a state hospital on a weekend pass, during which he hung himself in his parents' home.

He was, "an outlier." An outlier is a patient whose symptoms require more than an average amount of time to resolve.

When I mentioned, "outlier," to one peer reviewer he angrily responded that he was "a professor" with great experience and did not want to hear what I had to say.

To understand outlier, you have to understand statistics and the bell-shaped curve. Two thirds of people fall within one standard deviation of the average. Ninety five percent of people fall within two standard deviations of the average. Outliers fall more than two standard deviations from the average.

Acute care is treatment that is likely to result in functional recovery.

If the insurance company decides that ten days is the amount of time that ninety five percent of patients respond to during acute care, than it must accept the fact that two and one half percent of patients will require more than ten days of acute care.

I suspect that insurance companies do not give any of their customers more than the ten day authorization. That in my opinion is not right.

But who am I? I am just a doctor. I can be dropped from the panel. I can be bullied not to say anything.

On one occasion I announced to the peer reviewer that the conversation was on speaker phone and the patient was present and the peer reviewer became angry and flustered.

Something else I have noticed. Psychiatrists in hospitals tend to make daily changes in medications which tends to result in the patient receiving high doses of multiple medications in a short hospital stay.

This violates many of the best practices of psychiatry.

First of all, if the depression is exogenous and not endogenous, psychotherapy is indicated. Medications are not indicated.

If the patient has a chemical imbalance resulting in mania or depression, then medications are indicated.

If the patient is suddenly depressed and suicidal because of a loss of a job or separation or death, there is no chemical imbalance for the medications to correct.

Psychotherapy without medications is indicated. However, the lack of medications and medication changes is used as a basis for denial of additional days of treatment by the insurance company.

It is known the medications for depression take two to eight weeks to be effective. Denying hospital treatment for less than two weeks of treatment is not compatible with what is known about medications for depression and the proper treatment of depression.

The Peer to Peer review required by the insurance industry forces psychiatrists away from the best practices of psychiatry in order to keep the patient safe in the hospital until the patient is stable and safely treated outside of the hospital.

It is known that you have to increase medications for five or six patients for one patient to get better by virtue of the medication increase. This is called the Number Needed to Treat to get better, NNT to get better.

It is known that with each medication increase the patient is less likely to benefit and more likely to suffer injury from medication side effects.

The Number Needed to Treat to suffer harm is also referred to as the NNT to cause harm.

The number needed to treat to suffer harm, NNT to cause harm, gets smaller with each medication increase or addition.

With each increase or addition of medication the patient is less likely to obtain a benefit and more likely to suffer injury by side effect.

The notion that it is necessary to make frequent medication increases to justify "active treatment," and "authorize additional days of payment for hospital treatment," violates the best practices of psychiatry on many levels.

At this point the insurance industry joins hands with the pharmaceutical industry in applying pressure to the physician to prescribe high doses of multiple psychotropic medications.

Is this intentional or coincidental?

In both cases the focus is on the psychiatrist to prescribe medications and away from psychotherapy, which is expensive and labor intensive.

Psychotherapy for exogenous or reactive mental illness does not require psychotropic medications.

The best practice is the lowest effective dose of medications, not polypharmacy at high doses.

I was an expert witness for the Michigan Attorney General who was doing Medicaid Retroactive Audits of hospital admissions.

I received continuing medical education for doing these peer review audits. In 1993 I received 383 hours of continue education credits for peer review. In 1994 it was 253 hours. In 1995 it was 53 hours and in 1997 it was 5 hours of continuing education credits for peer review. I lost the letter for 1996.

After doing the peer review I was asked to testify in court during the Medicaid Retroactive Audits being conducted by the Michigan Attorney General.

In one case the admitting diagnosis was rectal digging. After about two years the discharge diagnosis was rectal digging. During the hospital stay it was determined that the patient was profoundly mentally retarded and had absolutely no language skills.

I testified that the daily group therapy and the hospital admission were not indicated. The condition was obviously chronic with no expectation of resolution with treatment.

The attorney examining me became distraught and asked if I was accusing his client of criminal activity.

I responded that I was retained to determine if the care was acute and appropriate for payment and I had determined that it was not.

I had not considered the possibility of criminal conduct, but if he wished, I could discuss the case through the lens of criminal conduct.

The attorney responded, "no," he did not wish me to discuss this case through the lens of criminal conduct and dismissed me as a witness.

The Michigan Attorney General chose not to ask me additional questions and I do not know what the resolution of that case was.

Before I went to Indiana, I interviewed for a position as a medical director of a "Stress Unit," in Marshall, Michigan.

A, "Stress Unit," is a fifteen or twenty bed psychiatric unit in a general hospital.

The unit was operated by PIA, Psychiatric Institutes of America, under contract with the general hospital.

The business manager advised me that I would be receiving a stipend to be the medical director and I would receive $5 for each day each patient was in the psychiatric hospital. That would be $75 dollars a day if there were fifteen patients in the hospital. In addition, I would be able to keep all the billing I submitted to the insurance companies for the patients I admitted and treated.

It never occurred to me that the $5 a day for each patient in the hospital was a problem. It was written into what they said was their standard contract. I assumed that a large corporation such as PIA had lawyers go over every contract.

I assumed that a large corporation such as PIA would make sure that they were in compliance with all of the rules and regulations that applied in each state they operated hospitals in.

However, the "Business of Medicine," approach of the business manager put me off. I elected to take the position of Medical Director of the Bowen Center in Warsaw, Indiana instead.

I knew that it would be more work and was farther from my children. However, it was more stable and I was more familiar with state agencies than with working for Corporate Medicine and the "Business of Medicine."

I wasn't being smart when I declined the job with PIA in Marshall, Michigan. I was lucky.

In 1993 a psychologist was sentenced to prison for accepting the $5 a day. It turns out that the $5 is called a kickback, or a bribe, for admitting patients to the hospital.

PIA was owned by National Medical Enterprises Inc. (NME).

NME was forced to divest itself of psychiatric hospitals and paid out many judgments over time in different courts.

In 1994 NME paid $379 million in fines and penalties to settle federal charges.

I suspect that the one psychologist went to jail so that the other psychiatrists and psychologists would line up with checkbooks in hand.

The rule is that "one who is liable must pay a

civil penalty of between $5,000 and $10,000 for each false claim (those amounts are adjusted from time to time; the current amounts are $5,500 to $11,000) and treble the amount of the government's damages."

If you admit one patient for three days and bill $100 dollars a day for three days of psychotherapy you are submitting three claims.

If these three claims are false claims, you owe the government $15,000 to $30,000 in fines and $900 in triple pay back for your original billing of $300.00 dollars.

If you have been doing this for ten years and had ten patients a day, you are looking at an entire career devoted to paying fines and penalties.

I was lucky. I decided not to take the job. I suppose that there are many psychiatrists paying fines and penalties for what they thought was just an ordinary business practice.

It would be interesting to have the GAO publish the total federal revenues from these lawsuits.

Medical school does not teach medical students

much about business or business law, etc.

Another face of the "Business of Medicine."

Hospital Corporation of America has another interesting face of business.

In 2002 HCA paid over $2 billion in restitutions, fines, and penalties.

What is interesting is the fact that Whistle blowers received substantial amounts.

An even more interesting fact is that there were Qui Tam lawsuits against HCA.

Qui Tam lawsuits are filed by private persons who collect a percentage of the revenues.

If anyone attempts to defraud the government there is a possibility of being a whistleblower and collecting a percentage of the fines and penalties or filing a Qui Tam lawsuit under the False Claims Act (FCA), 31 U.S.C. §§ 3729 – 3733.

"If the government intervenes in the qui tam action, the relator is entitled to receive between 15 and 25 percent of the amount recovered by the government through the qui tam action."

"If the government declines to intervene in the action, the relator's share is increased to 25 to 30 percent. "

I suppose a disgruntled employee has given, "the business ," to the "Business of Medicine," in more than one instance.

I read that one whistle blower received ten percent of $100,000,000 or $10,000,000.

In 1993 I read an article that stated that the total income of all of the physicians in the United States was $10,000,000,000, (ten billion dollars).

The article also stated that in 1993 the medical insurance company profits were about $100,000,000,000 (one hundred billion dollars).

The article stated that doctors attempted to contract with employers to split the $100,000,000,000 of insurance company profits between the doctors and employers. The employers would save $50,000,000,000 and the doctors would gain $50,000,000,000.

The insurance industry used their $100,000,000,000 in profits to lobby in Washington DC, the state capitals and the press to make it an antitrust violation for medical doctors to compete with the insurance industry.

The insurance industry used the $100,000,000.000 in profits to make doctors look like greedy pigs in the press. Needless to say, the insurance industry won.

Are doctors greedy pigs? Are insurance companies greedy, rapacious pigs? Do no harm?

Since 2008 I have been a contractor. I sign up with a recruiter and pay part of my salary to the recruiter for the privilege of working with the recruiter's client.

For example, if the recruiter has a client the client pays the recruiter $200 for every hour I work.

The recruiter pays me $160 dollars for every hour I work and keeps $40 for every hour I work.

I can be dismissed without notice and I can quit without notice. I receive no health insurance. I receive a rental car, malpractice insurance and temporary housing during the period of the work assignment.

I do not know how much the recruiter is being paid. I do not know what their profit is.

I do know that I am paying for the privilege of working.

When I was growing up, I drank water from a garden hose and never thought of paying for water.

When I was growing up, employees belonged to unions

When I was growing up, employees had medical insurance, pensions and paid vacations and I did not know anyone that paid for the privilege of working.

The world has changed. The new "Business of Medicine" is that hospitals make a profit off the work of doctors and doctors pay for the privilege of working.

I have been paying for the privilege of working since 2008 at about twenty different assignments.

I know that in 1984 I left about $250,000 dollars of uncollected billing when I left private practice. I do not know how much I have been paying for the privilege of working since 2008 as a contracting psychiatrist.

Recently I was offered a salary of about $300,000 salary to work with three other psychiatrists at an eighty-bed facility. The salary did not allow for payment for hours worked past forty hours a week. The doctor is required to treat all twenty patients, even if it is more than forty hours a week. I declined.

That is twenty beds per psychiatrists.

I believe that there should be a psychiatrist for every twelve psychiatric beds. It takes about an hour to do an initial evaluation, sometimes an hour and a half, depending upon the patient's willingness to cooperate.

It takes about an hour to do the discharge paperwork.

If the average length of stay is three days that means, four admissions a day, four discharges a day and four daily rounds a day. That is a minimum of nine hours a day.

The notion that a severely mentally ill patient can be adequately treated in three days is based upon insurance companies and their reluctance to pay for necessary services.

If the attending physician routinely discharges based upon prior authorization denials he is allowing the insurance company to practice medicine with his license. Integrity? Money? The patient?

Recently I quit a job because it was too much work to manage a twelve bed psychiatric unit, and also be the only psychiatrist doing consultations and the only psychiatrist covering a busy emergency room.

The "Business of Medicine," is now the business of, "Doctor Burnout."

How many billable hours can you squeeze out of a doctor if you are a hospital and the doctor is on salary?

How complex and detailed can you make the billing process so that you can maximize the opportunity to deny payment if you are the insurance company?

How much money can you demand in payback after retrospective audits of billing under the claim that a hospital admission was not necessary?

Let me summarize the situation for the practicing doctor.

The doctor can expect either to pay for his job or have the hospital as employer make a profit from the doctor's revenue stream.

The doctor can expect to work more than forty hours a week.

The doctor can be expected to spend many hours doing tediously detailed documentation to acquire payment from insurance companies.

The insurance company grants prior authorization for the hospital admission and treatment.

The insurance company conducts retrospective audits and demands part of past payment back on an annual audit.

Now let us look at medical care through the lens of the patient.

The patient has to choose a doctor from a panel of doctors. The panel can change from year to year. The insurance company can eliminate the most expensive doctors and replace them every year.

The expensive doctors are the doctors that order lab tests, consultations, expensive medicines and hospital admissions.

The patient can ask. "did I get the cheap medication because the doctor was afraid of being dropped from the panel?

"Was I denied surgery because the doctor was afraid of being dropped from the panel?"

"Did the doctor fail to order a neurology consultation, a psychiatric consultation, a cardiology consultation because the doctor was afraid of being dropped from the panel?"

"Did the doctor order my medication because the other medication was not in the formulary provided by the insurance company?"

"During my hospital admission did the doctor order my medication because the other medication was not in the hospital formulary?"

The standard of care is informed choice. The doctor diagnoses the medical condition and explains the risks and the benefits of the choices to the patient.

The patient then makes a choice among the risks and the benefits.

The patient and doctor are not alone. In the room with the patient and the doctor is the medical policy. That policy is written by attorneys and actuaries employed by the insurance company.

The trade secrets are not made explicit in the insurance policy. The trade secrets that give the insurance company the competitive edge are how costs are controlled after the medical insurance is purchased.

The average length of stay allowed by the peer to peer call can be a trade secret.

The basis for retrospective audits can be a trade secret.

The basis for selecting and removing physicians from panels approved to bill for medical services can be a trade secret.

The lawyers, the actuaries, and the trade secrets are invisible, but present in every transaction between the doctor and the patient.

The patient might wonder why his doctor from last year is not his doctor this year. That is probably a trade secret.

This essay is an introduction to a very complex situation. A full understanding will require many hours of additional research on the part of the reader.

This is just the tip of the ice burg.

I cannot put a lifetime if experience into fifty or sixty pages of text.

If I am put on the stand to testify, I don't know what I would say. It would depend upon how the questions were framed.

"Preexisting text," includes names of corporations, names of law cases, and text of statutes cited including but not limited to "Qui Tam lawsuit under the False Claims Act (FCA), 31 U.S.C. §§ 3729 – 3733."

My copyright claim is a clam to the "original text," which is my commentary on the corporations, the law cases, and text of statutes and my personal experiences as reported in this essay presented as a psychiatric consultation to the general public.

Patient Satisfaction and Dr. Burnout
The Long View
Your 22nd Psychiatric Consultation
William R. Yee M.D., J.D.
Copyright applied for March 14, 2021

Introduction

Recently I was advised that there were a series of patients reporting dissatisfaction with my treatment.

I was not given the patient's names or the basis for their dissatisfaction.

All I knew is that one patient had reported to a therapist that she was dissatisfied with my treatment because I would not prescribe Lunesta.

This could be any of my patients because I inform all my patients on the first visit that I do not prescribe addicting medications because like all facilities, all neighborhoods there is an epidemic of alcoholism and drug addiction.

Lunesta is addicting and has the additional FDA warning against next day drowsiness.

I rely on:

[5-15-2014] The U.S. Food and Drug
Administration (FDA) is warning that the
insomnia drug Lunesta (eszopiclone) can cause
next-day impairment of driving and other
activities that require alertness. As a result,
we have decreased the recommended starting
dose of Lunesta to 1 mg at bedtime. Health
care professionals should follow the new dosing
recommendations when starting patients on
Lunesta. Patients should continue taking their
prescribed dose of Lunesta and contact their
health care professionals to ask about the most
appropriate dose for them.

FDA Drug Safety Communication: FDA warns
of next-day impairment with the sleep aid
Lunesta (eszopiclone) and lowers recommended
dose.

Because any medication can cause drowsiness
the next day, on the first contact I give all my
patients a written handout that states that if
the patient is drowsy while driving a police
officer can give them a ticket for impaired

driving under the influence of the medication. I also give patients written advice that the officer may see small children in the car and be required to report to Child Protective Services to put the children into Foster Care.

Lunesta, and the other Z Drugs all have the following FDA warning:

FDA adds Boxed Warning for risk of serious injuries caused by sleepwalking with certain prescription insomnia medicines.

FDA Drug Safety Communication

"[04-30-2019] The Food and Drug Administration (FDA) is advising that rare but serious injuries have happened with certain common prescription insomnia medicines because of sleep behaviors, including sleepwalking, sleep driving, and engaging in other activities while not fully awake. These complex sleep behaviors have also resulted in deaths. These behaviors appear to be more common with eszopiclone (Lunesta), zaleplon (Sonata), and zolpidem (Ambien, Ambien CR, Edluar, Intermezzo, Zolpimist) than other prescription medicines used for sleep."

"As a result, we are requiring a Boxed Warning, our most prominent warning, to be added to the prescribing information and the patient Medication Guides for these medicines. We are also requiring a Contraindication, our strongest warning, to avoid use in patients who have previously experienced an episode of complex sleep behavior with eszopiclone, zaleplon, and zolpidem."

The Long View: My Fifty Years

My medical education started in 1968 at the age of twenty-one.

I attended Bible School at the age of four and learned the Golden Rule, treat others the way you would have them treat you.

I am Chinese and Swedish and multicultural by DNA and family environment.

My favorite class in college was a class in Social Anthropology that explored the many ways that different cultures manage child rearing, marriage, social relationships, law and other cultural issues.

After completing medical school, I swore the Hippocratic Oath to do no harm.

In training as a psychiatric resident, I was educated in psychoanalysis including the concepts of transference, countertransference, and resistance to treatment.

I was trained in Freudian analysis, Jungian analysis, Rogerian analysis, Adlerian analysis, Horneyian analysis, etc.

I learned about the oral, anal, phallic, latent, and genital stages of psychosexual development of maturation from birth to adult life.

I learned about unconditional positive regard from the Rogerian school of psychoanalysis

I learned about birth order, social and cultural issues from Alfred Adler's school of psychoanalysis.

I learned about women's issues from Karen Horney's school of psychoanalysis.

I learned about social issues from Erich

Fromm's school of psychoanalysis.

Medical ethics requires that:

1. I respect the patient
2. I listen to the patient
3. I am transparent with the patent
4. I educate the patient
5. I promote patient autonomy

What does medical ethics mean in practice?

Respect means that I make accommodations to the patient's culture, gender, and preferences.

I ask patients if they want a chaperone, the door open or closed, if they want counseling, medication, or both. How often they want to be seen, if they have suggestions for improving service, if they are satisfied with treatment, when they want to see me next. It is always the patient's choice.

Listening to the patient is more perception than reality.

To accommodate patients' perceptions, I ask them if they want me type their words into the note word for word as they speak, or if they want me to write a summary after the face-to-face meeting is completed.

Some patients have the perception that I am not listening to them even though I am typing their statements word for word into the progress note.

Other patients prefer that I type their statements word for word into the progress notes because they do not want any distortions of their statements to be part of the medical record.

You can have one, but not both, unless you tape record the interview. Unfortunately, I do not have the equipment to tape record my interviews with the patients.

I am transparent with the patient. I advise the patient as to my role.

6. I am an expert witness for the court.
7. I am an expert witness for the plaintiff.
8. I am an expert witness for the defendants.

9. I am the personal physician of the patient.
10. I have obligations to report child abuse to child protective services.
11. I have obligations to report crimes to various authorities.
12. I have obligations to report threats to various authorities.
13. I offer medications that reduce symptoms by 20% to 40% on average in one out of every three or four patients treated.
14. I advise the patient that more than fifty percent of patients stop taking medications or don't fill their prescriptions for medications.
15. I rarely cure mental illness and I cannot refer the patient to a psychiatrist who usually cures mental illness.
16. I recommend meditation, aerobic exercise, sleep hygiene, meditation, deep breathing, relaxation, stimulus desensitization, EMDR, Cognitive behavior therapy and other alternatives before starting medications.
17. I recommend that the medications are started at a low dose to minimize side effects.

18. I recommend that the medications be titrated up slowly to allow for the body to adjust to the medication side effect.
19. I recommend that the medication be used only as a temporary treatment until symptoms are adequately controlled by alternative treatments or remit.
20. I advise the patient that I will start the medications with or without alternative treatments after advising the patient to exhaust the alternatives first.
21. It remains the patient's decision whether or not to take medications.
22. It remains my duty to educate the patient as to the risks and benefits of alternative treatments.
23. I will offer one medication after another until the patient has had the opportunity to try them all or feels that medications are a waste of time.

Medication noncompliance is greater than fifty percent and is 75% according to some research.

I rely on

Pediatric Psychotropic Medication Compliance:
Page 67 of 178

A Literature Review and Research-Based Suggestions for Improving Treatment Compliance
Sabine Hack and Byron Chow
Journal of Child and Adolescent PsychopharmacologyVol. 11, No. 1Articles Published Online:5 Jul 2004https://doi.org/10.1089/104454601750143465

And

Psychotropic medication non-adherence and its associated factors among patients with major psychiatric disorders: a systematic review and meta-analysis
Agumasie Semahegn, Kwasi Torpey, Adom Manu,1 Nega Assefa, Gezahegn Tesfaye, and Augustine Ankomah
Syst Rev. 2020; 9: 17.
Published online 2020 Jan 16. doi: 10.1186/s13643-020-1274-3
PMCID: PMC6966860
PMID: 31948489

On the first face to face appointment, I give the patient a six-page printout about the treatments of mental illness.

This is because there is too much information to remember and not enough time according to current practices in brief therapy.

I promote patient autonomy.

At every point it is the patient's choice:

24. Do you want a chaperone?
25. Do you want the door opened or closed?
26. Do you want me to type every word you speak or write a summary after the face-to-face appointment is completed?
27. Do you want psychotherapy, medication, or both?
28. Do you want to see me weekly or on some other schedule?
29. Do you have suggestions on how I can improve my services?

I have been the medical director of two mental health centers.

I have done annual performance evaluations of residents in training, medical doctors, and psychiatrists under my supervision.

Evidence- based medicine is the Gold Standard

of Medical Care.

In medicine, and particularly in psychiatry, evidenced based medicine is an imaginary construct because the research is of low quality and not reproducible

The dilemma of annual performance evaluations is that science does not provide tools for performance evaluation beyond attendance and completion of paperwork.

I rely on:

1,500 scientists lift the lid on reproducibility
Survey sheds light on the 'crisis' rocking research.
Monya Baker
NATURE | NEWS FEATURE
25 May 2016 Corrected: 28 July 2016

And

Bad papers are still published. But some other things might be getting better.
By Kelsey Piper Oct 14, 2020, 12:20pm EDT

As a medical director I was confronted with this dilemma.

If I gave a substandard performance evaluation, I was admitting that I could not hire competent psychiatrists and doctors.

If I gave a substandard performance evaluation, I was admitting that I could not train medical students, psychiatric residents, doctors, and psychiatrists that had been successful all their lives until they came under my supervision.

To make things worse the weakness in research did not offer me tools for training or performance evaluation that are evidenced based.

Let us explore the psychiatric research to examine the state of the art on March 13th, 2021.

This research has the goal of determining what the physician can do to improve patient satisfaction.

The converse is to identify physician behaviors

that contribute to patient dissatisfaction.

There are many studies examining the basis for patient satisfaction.

These studies have been inconclusive and offer contradictory results that invalidate any claim that patient satisfaction is based upon specific factors.

The research on patient satisfaction does not support any sound basis for determining the cause of patient satisfaction and patient dissatisfaction.

The operant fact is that person-related characteristics have been found to be both determinants and confounders simultaneously and not reliable as a basis of determining the basis for patient satisfaction and dissatisfaction.

I rely on:

Determinants of patient satisfaction: a systematic review
Enkhjargal Batbaatar, Javkhlanbayar Dorjdagva, Ariunbat Luvsannyam, Matteo

Mario Savino, Pietro Amenta
A Perspect Public Health 2017 Mar;137(2):89-
101. doi: 10.1177/1757913916634136. Epub
2016 Jul 20.
PMID: 27004489 DOI:
10.1177/1757913916634136

Patient safety and clinical effectiveness are
positively related to patient satisfaction which
is not related to characteristics of the
physician.

I rely on:

A systematic review of evidence on the links
between patient experience and clinical safety
and effectiveness
Cathal Doyle1, Laura Lennox1,2, Derek Bell1,2
Published by the BMJ Publishing Group
Limited.
Volume 3, Issue 1

The operant thought in this article is that
patient satisfaction is an imaginary construct
without validity on a scientific basis. The basis
of patient satisfaction remains to be identified
by research and remains debatable.

I rely on:

A systematic review of patient and caregivers' satisfaction with telehealth videoconferencing as a mode of service delivery in managing patients' health

Joseph F. Orlando ,
Matthew Beard ,
Saravana Kumar
Published: August 30, 2019
https://doi.org/10.1371/journal.pone.0221848

My experience is that doctor burnout is a product of increasing the patient caseload, increasing the documentation requirements, and reducing the time available to complete the assigned tasks.

This is a universal experience in all employment situations to reduce costs and increase cash flow. This is a simple equation.

In the article below Burnout was defined by the following factors:

1. overall burnout
2. emotional exhaustion

3. depersonalization

4. personal accomplishment

Associated with physician burnout were:

1. depression and

2. emotional distress

The operant work products of physician
burnout are:

1. unprofessional behaviors

2. unsafe care

3. low patient satisfaction

4. depersonalization

What is unprofessional behavior?

Professionalism and unprofessionalism are to
sides of the same coin and subject to many
definitions by many writers.

The article below adopts four abstract concepts
which are also subject to various definitions
and therefore remain artificial constructs. They
are:

1. excellence

2. accountability

3. altruism
4. humanism

As these are abstract concepts professionalism was further defined by the following factors to approximate professionalism:

1. adherence to treatment guidelines
2. referrals to treatment or other services
3. malpractice claims
4. poor communication practices
5. low empathy

What is low patient satisfaction?

1. Patient reported satisfaction and
2. perceived enablement scores

What is depersonalization? The authors below relied on the Maslach Burnout Inventory™ (MBI) to define depersonalization:

1. lack of empathy
   a. Unfeeling engagement with the patient
   b. impersonal engagement with the patient

While being trained in psychoanalysis the psychiatrist is trained to be neutral in response to avoid shaping the patient's thoughts and feelings. It can be argued that by giving positive responses the psychiatrist is molded into a codependent in prolonging the illness. The positive responses by the psychiatrist can be experienced as a reward for being mentally ill, thereby prolonging the mental illness through positive reinforcement.

If a facility has a common problem with protracting and enhancing mental illness such as PTSD, then it is incumbent upon the facility to look at the corporate culture and what common factors enhance and prolong the PTSD.

I rely on:

Association Between Physician Burnout and Patient Safety, Professionalism, and Patient Satisfaction
A Systematic Review and Meta-analysis
Maria Panagioti, PhD; Keith Geraghty, PhD; Judith Johnson, PhD; et al, Anli Zhou, MD; Efharis Panagopoulou, PhD; Carolyn Chew-Graham, MD; David Peters, MD; Alexander Hodkinson, PhD; Ruth Riley, PhD; Aneez Esmail, MD, PhD

Original Investigation Physician Work
Environment and Well-Being
September 4, 2018
JAMA Intern Med. 2018;178(10):1317-1331.
doi:10.1001/jamainternmed.2018.3713

Although research on Team Based Care reveals
some benefit. The suboptimal quality of
research requires better research to confirm
and clarify the actual benefits and costs.

I rely on:

Can Team-Based Care Improve Patient
Satisfaction? A Systematic Review of
Randomized Controlled Trials
July 2014PLoS ONE 9(7):e100603
DOI: 10.1371/journal.pone.0100603
Source Pub Med

Now let us examine patient dissatisfaction.

Patient dissatisfaction is associated (caused?)
by the following:
1. ineptitude
2. disrespect
3. waits
4. ineffective communication

5. lack of environmental control
6. substandard amenities (6.9%).

I rely on

What can we learn from patient dissatisfaction? An analysis of dissatisfying events at an academic medical center
By: Alicia V. Lee, MD, John P. Moriarty, MD, Christopher Borgstrom, Leora I. Horwitz, MD, MHS
J. Hosp. Med. 2010 November;5(9):514-520 | 10.1002/jhm.861

Politics can be an issue among medical staffs in various organizations.

Political skills are as important as medical skills.

Is building your brand important? The following four attributes are important in a medical career:
1. likability
2. achievements
3. connections/friend at work
4. political skills.

I rely on:

Hospital Politics Don't Have to Be a Dirty Business
MICHAEL SILVERMAN, MD and DREW WHITE, MD, MBA ON OCTOBER 10, 2017
Copyright © 2019 EPMonthly.com

I suppose the takeaway is that the physician must
1. keep up with his medical education with Continuing Medical Education to maintain licensing and medical staff appointments.
2. Sustain political activities to maintain his brand among the medical staff.

Who determines which physician is "problematic" in the Medical Staff?

Is it the:
30. Hospital CEO?
31. Hospital Executive Committee?
32. Hospital Peer Review Committee?
33. Chief of the Medical Staff?
34. Departmental Chairmen?
35. Medical Staff Peer?
36. Anonymous Other?

Since politics are a part of every medical staff there are many issues that may start the process of reviewing a physician for "problematic," behavior.

There are many issues that make a Medical Staff Member, "problematic":

37. Criminal Behaviors.
38. Drug and Alcohol abuse.
39. Abuse of Staff and Patients.
40. Whistle blowing.
41. Patient complaints and low satisfaction ratings.
42. Cultural Differences in practice style.
43. Eccentric Documentation.
44. Eccentric Referral Patterns.

Hospitals, Medical Staffs, and Medical Staff Members have created problems for themselves by "corrective actions," addressing the, "problematic physician." The following are some of the problems based upon my personal experience and review of the literature:

45. Lawsuits with money judgments for wrongful termination.
46. Lawsuits with money judgments for defamation.

47. Lawsuits with money judgments for violation of 42 U.S. Code § 1983;
48. Lawsuits with money judgments for violation of 42 U.S. Code § 1985;
49. Hospital records seized by United States Marshals and made public records.
50. Prosecution for criminal activities.
51. Subjected to additional reviews by the Joint Commission.
52. Loss of Joint Commission Accreditation.
53. Bad press and loss of community confidence.
54. Congressional investigations and interventions.
55. Change of Facility Chain of Command from the CEO on down.
56. Loss of immunities for failure to comply with statutory time limits.

The Health Care Quality Improvement Act of 1986 -H.R.5540 — 99th Congress (1985-1986) was designed to provide guidelines for managing medical staff, protecting medical staff rights and offering immunities for the medical facility managing medical staff in "good faith."

Let us dissect the following:

"Provides protection from liability under Federal and State laws for members of a professional review body and their staffs who, in the reasonable belief that the action was in the furtherance of quality health care, warranted by the facts known, and after a reasonable effort to obtain the facts, take actions which adversely affect the clinical privileges or professional society membership of a physician. Provides such protection to those who provide information to professional review bodies."

The physician subject to an adverse action by the "professional review body and their staffs"

What is the professional review body?

The physician's attorney will argue that the "professional review body" includes, but is not limited to:

57. The Facility CEO
58. The Facility Executive Committee
59. The Facility Pharmacy Committee
60. The Facility Credentialing Committee
61. The Facility Peer Review Committee
62. The Facility Medical Records Committee
63. The Physician's supervisor

64. The chain of command between the Physician's supervisor and the CEO
65. Any other Facility employee or officer that intersects the physician and that physician's activity at the Facility.

Let us dissect the concept of reasonable belief. What is a "Reasonable Belief?"

The physician's attorney will want to know what are the facts that form the "reasonable belief?"

66. Who alleged that the physician's conduct was defective?
67. What was the allegation?
68. What was the motivation for making the allegation?
69. Did the person who made the allegation have a history of other allegations?
70. Were there similar allegations by others?
71. When was the physician notified of the defective conduct?
72. What was the physician's response to the allegation?
73. Which individual or Committee investigated the allegation?
74. What are in the records of that investigation?

Let us dissect, "the reasonable belief," that are warranted by the facts known:

The attorney for the physician will want to know:

75. "What is the reasonable belief," that supports your action?
76. What are the facts that support your, "reasonable belief?"
77. What are alternative "reasonable beliefs," based upon these facts?
78. What were the physician's stated reasonable beliefs?
79. What was your basis for not accepting the physician's "reasonable belief"?

Let us examine "furtherance of quality health care,"

80. How does your "reasonable belief," serve the best interest of the facility, patients, and the affected physician?
81. What are viable alternative "reasonable beliefs"?
82. How do the alternative "reasonable beliefs" serve the best interest of the facility, patients, and the affected Physician?

Let us dissect "reasonable effort to obtain the facts":

83. What did you do to obtain the facts?
84. When did you make the effort to obtain the facts?
85. When did you contact the affected physician?
86. What did you tell the affected physician?
87. What was the affected physician's response?
88. What was your effort to confirm the affected physician's response?
89. In what ways were your efforts different from prior practice?
90. Is there a possibility that the allegations were mistaken?
91. Is there a possibility that the allegations were false?
92. Are you convinced that your investigation was thorough and without bias of any kind?

Let us dissect the actions taken that adversely affect the clinical privileges or professional society membership?
1. How were similar allegations against other physicians managed?

2. What corrective actions were offered to the physician?
3. When were the corrective actions offered to the physician?
4. What were the alternative actions available to the individual or committee?
5. Why was the action taken rather than the alternative actions?
6. What was the practice with prior physicians in regard to corrective actions?
7. Are you sure you eliminated all bias in these proceedings?
8. Are you sure that you took the best possible course of action?

I rely on my personal experience and the following for addressing "problematic behaviors above:

Medical Staff Management Can Be Minefield
 August 1, 2017
© 2021 Relias. All rights reserved.

Patient Satisfaction and Patient Complaints: The Long View, My 50 Years

Let us look at patient complaints. Based upon my fifty years of practice and researching the literature patient complaints can be based upon:

93. Personal Preference
94. Mistake
95. Mental Illness
96. Munchhausen Disorder
97. Secondary Gain
98. Criminal Behavior
99. Sport

Personal Preference:

Often the patient does not want the physician to be completing a progress note in the computer during the fact to face appointment. Other patients want their statement entered into the record word for word as they speak to avoid distortion by memory.

I now make the following offer to the patient:

Do you want me to type your statements word

for word while we take, or do you want me to take short notes and type a summary after the face-to-face meeting is completed?

The patient will choose between the following to statements for the record:

"I want my words typed into the note exactly as stated while we talk."

or:

"I want you to take short notes while we talk and write a brief summary after the face-to-face appointment is over."

Memories are reconstructed constructs and prone to error.

Patients often record doctor visits without the doctor's knowledge.

Federal law allows patients to tape record meetings without the doctor's knowledge. I always assume the patient is tape recording the meeting as it will not alter my treatment and I cannot search them for recording devices without their consent.

Surgeons have videotaped the patient giving consent to surgery including reviewing the risks and indicating that they understand the risk and accept the risks of the surgical procedure. They do this to avoid errors on the part of the patient and the physician based upon reconstructed memories.

I rely on:

The fallibility of memory in judicial processes: Lessons from the past and their modern consequences
Mark L. Howe, and Lauren M. Knott
Memory. 2015 Jul 4; 23(5): 633–656.
Published online 2015 Feb 23. doi: 10.1080/09658211.2015.1010709
PMCID: PMC4409058
PMID: 25706242

Complaints based upon mental illness.

The most famous case of complaints based upon mental illness is The McMartin preschool trial. The McMartin preschool trial was based upon sexual abuse case in the 1980s.

The McMartin preschool trial was based upon a false complaint by a woman who suffered from paranoid schizophrenia.

False complaints based upon mental illness are common in mental health facilities.

I worked a State Hospital in Kalamazoo Michigan where false allegations were made almost daily, but each one was formally investigated by the State Police as required by law.

Complaints based upon secondary gain.

Patients will make complaints against the physician because:

1.. They are addicted to drugs and alcohol and the physician refuses to prescribe addictive medications such as Xanax or Lunesta.

2.. The patient wants disability benefits, and the physician does not find a disability.

3.. The patient is subjective to criminal prosecution and the physician does not find the patient mentally incompetent to stand trial or insane to avoid conviction.

4..The patient wants addicting medications for resale and the physician refuses to prescribe addicting medications for chronic symptoms.

5..The patient wants time off from work and the physician does not find a basis to grant time off from work for medical reasons.

6.. Other reasons based upon divorce proceedings, child custody issues, lawsuits disputing wills, etc.

Complaints based upon criminal activities:

When I was working for the Michigan Department of Corrections from 1987 to 1991, they had a course entitled, "Anatomy of a Setup."

Anatomy of a Setup taught employees for the Michigan Department of Corrections how inmates would work as teams to trick a naive employee into making a series of rule violations. Then inmates would convince the employee that if they did not bring in drugs and engage in sex with the inmates the inmates would report the employee who would be prosecuted and go to prison.

This was not an idle threat as it is well known that prisoners have bribed employees into bringing drugs. The employees were then caught, prosecuted, and incarcerated.

In Michigan, the "Anatomy of a Setup," was taught by correctional officers who were trapped, but reported their issues to their superiors. They were not fired. They became credible trainers in the Anatomy of a Setup.

There are many reasons that a criminal will make false complaints or make threats of false complaints against physicians. Violence against health care workers is a crime, but rarely prosecuted.

I rely on:

Prevalence and policy of occupational violence against oral healthcare workers: systematic review and meta-analysis.
Binmadi, N.O., Alblowi, J.A.
BMC Oral Health 19, 279 (2019).
https://doi.org/10.1186/s12903-019-0974-3

Let us examine, "good faith," in making a record that supports a corrective action against a physician.

The U.S. Equal Employment Opportunity Commission, which was established by Title VII of the Civil Rights Act of 1964

The Civil Rights Act of 1964 prohibits discrimination and harassment of any type and affords equal employment opportunities to employees and applicants without regard to race, color, religion, sex, sexual orientation, gender identity or expression, pregnancy, age, national origin, disability status, genetic information, protected.

The United States Department of State has the following as a part of its policy:

"Any employee who believes he or she has been the target of sexual harassment is encouraged to inform the offending person orally or in writing that such conduct is unwelcome and offensive and must stop."

Why is this a policy?

The answer is that employees have encouraged a pattern of social conduct and then file a complaint. This is known as "entrapment."

The United State Department of Justice Defines Entrapment as:

645. ENTRAPMENT—ELEMENTS

Entrapment is a complete defense to a criminal charge, on the theory that "Government agents may not originate a criminal design, implant in an innocent person's mind the disposition to commit a criminal act, and then induce commission of the crime so that the Government may prosecute." Jacobson v. United States, 503 U.S. 540, 548 (1992). A valid entrapment defense has two related elements: (1) government inducement of the crime, and (2) the defendant's lack of predisposition to engage in the criminal conduct. Mathews v. United States, 485 U.S. 58, 63 (1988). Of the two elements, predisposition is by far the more important.

Inducement is the threshold issue in the entrapment defense. Mere solicitation to commit a crime is not inducement. Sorrells v.

United States, 287 U.S. 435, 451 (1932). Nor does the government's use of artifice, stratagem, pretense, or deceit establish inducement. Id. at 441. Rather, inducement requires a showing of at least persuasion or mild coercion, United States v. Nations, 764 F.2d 1073, 1080 (5th Cir. 1985); pleas based on need, sympathy, or friendship, ibid.; or extraordinary promises of the sort "that would blind the ordinary person to his legal duties," United States v. Evans, 924 F.2d 714, 717 (7th Cir. 1991). See also United States v. Kelly, 748 F.2d 691, 698 (D.C. Cir. 1984) (inducement shown only if government's behavior was such that "a law-abiding citizen's will to obey the law could have been overborne"); United States v. Johnson, 872 F.2d 612, 620 (5th Cir. 1989) (inducement shown if government created "a substantial risk that an offense would be committed by a person other than one ready to commit it").

It is a tedious and uncertain task to prove or disprove "entrapment."

The obligation to object to "offensive behaviors," simplifies the process because behavior persisting after the notice is indicative of intent without inducement.

This obligation of notice with continuation of "problematic conduct" without corrective action is a factor in good faith.

If there is no notice with the opportunity of a good faith corrective action, it is difficult to support the assertion of good faith in applying any corrective action.

If there is no notice of "problematic behavior," with opportunity to make a corrective action there is insufficient basis to assert adequate training and supervision.

The issue of adequate training and supervision is an issue that allows the supervisor and the annual performance evaluation, the Executive Committee, the Credentialing Committee, the Chief of the Medical Staff, the Pharmaceutical Committee, the CEO and any other agent of the Medical Facility to be named as defendant for wrongful termination, libel, slander and a host of Complaints to be filed by the attorney with a fertile mind.

I have had patients that were the wives and children of police officers, ministers, psychiatrists, psychologists, and social workers.

Police officers, ministers, psychiatrists, psychologists, and social workers are preoccupied with good and evil and doing the right thing in difficult circumstances.

The children of these people often like to provoke their parents by breaking the law, sinning, violating social norms and even putting a tattoo of the bar code used in the jail during a period of incarceration on public display.

I had a lady bring her minister in for joint psychotherapy. What was peculiar was that the patient had no anxiety, anger, or depression. On the contrary the minister was very uncomfortable, and the patient was euphoric. I did not understand what was going on, but it just didn't seem right.

Later the minister was in the news for having sexual contact with a member of his ministry.

It all became clear. The practice of psychiatry is never simple or predictable.

This is merely an introduction to the many issues that intersect the concept of patient satisfaction.

This missive must end at some time and I choose to end it here.

I am here to do no harm and help if I can.

Thank you for your time and attention.

William R. Yee M.D., J.D.
Board Certified Psychiatrist.
Practicing Medicine and Psychiatry without interruption since 1972 in Michigan, Indiana, Kentucky, California, and Texas
Recently licensed in Texas and excited about opportunities to live and practice in Texas, at your service.

"Pre-Existing text," includes names of symptoms, medical illnesses, medications, people, corporations, agencies, law cases, text of law cases, statutes, text of statutes, policies, the text of policies, the titles of articles, of books, the content of articles and books cited.

My copyright claim is a clam to the "original text," which is my personal experiences as described in the text above and my commentary on the names of symptoms, medical illnesses, medications, people, names of agencies, corporations, law cases, text of law cases, statutes, text of statutes, policies, the text of policies, the titles of articles, of books, the content of articles and books cited.

Bullying, Burnout, or Moral Injury? The
Many Faces of Democide
Your 28th Psychiatric Consultation
William R. Yee M.D., J.D.
Copyright Applied for 01/09/22

Introduction: Democide

The reader will better understand the
substance of this missive if the reader
understands the context.

First, the reader should understand what
Democide is.

Democide is the murder of citizens by the
government. Democide is pervasive in
government.

Governments kill their own citizens to assert
power. Socrates is an example of selective
democide.

Socrates, born 470 years before the birth of
Christ in Athens, Greece and died 399 years
before the birth of Christ in Athens Greece.
Socrates was an ancient Greek philosopher

whose life and thought profoundly influences Western philosophy.

I suggest reading,
The Hemlock Cup: Socrates, Athens and the Search for the Good Life, February 14, 2012, by Bettany Hughes.

Socrates was murdered by his own government because he threatened the power of a few individuals in the government.

Socrates is an example of Old Wisdom, "No good deed goes unpunished."

Socrates is an example of the Butterfly Effect.

Each of us has the power by simply talking to create a huge and long-lasting effect on the future of the World.

Your few words here and there can create another Butterfly Effect that changes the course of history.

For want of a nail the horse lacked a shoe.
For want of a shoe the soldier lacked a horse.
For want of a horse the cavalry lacked a man.

For want of a man the cavalry lost the battle.
For want of that battle the empire lost the war.
For want of a victory in the war the empire fell
into ruins and was forgotten in the pages of
history.

Rummel estimated that there have been 262
million victims of democide in the 20th
century, From Wikipedia, the free
encyclopedia.

Genghis Khan is responsible for the Mongol
Empire, and one estimate is that about 11% of
the world's population was killed either during
or immediately after the Mongol invasions
(around 37.75–60 million people)
https://en.wikipedia.org/wiki/Destruction_unde
r_the_Mongol_Empire.

At some point conquerors become rulers and
murder of citizens persists after war to sustain
power and control.

Self-Organizing Systems
Another way of looking at government is
through the lens of self-organizing systems.
Self-organizing systems are elements that
interact according to a few simple rules in a

manner that presents with the appearance of order and organization.

Self-organization occurs in many physical, chemical, biological, robotic, and cognitive systems.

Examples of self-organization include crystallization, thermal convection of fluids, chemical oscillation, animal swarming, neural circuits, and black markets.
From Wikipedia, the free encyclopedia.

Politics, the stock market, and most social organizations fall into the category of self-organizing systems.

The order is an illusion and allows for short term predictability that evaporates in attempts at long term predictability.

Attempts to maintain order are eventually defeated in strange and unpredictable ways.

An example is the fall of any empire or the fall of the Berlin Wall

I suggest as an introduction to this topic:

Emergence: The Connected Lives of Ants, Brains, Cities, and Software by Steven Johnson
Paperback – September 10, 2002
Politics, the weather, the stock market, businesses, governments, and medical facilities are examples of self-organizing systems. Chaos theory describes the mathematics of these systems.

Chaos Theory
Chaos theory rests in nonlinear equations. A linear equation has one unknown, any number of constants, and is limited to a power of one,

e.g., $X = bY + a$ where b and a are constants and the only unknown is the Y

A nonlinear equation has more than one unknown, and a power of 2 or more with any number of constants.
e.g., $X = aY^2 + bZ + c$
Where Y is an unknown to the power of 2 and Z is an unknown and a, b, and c are constants.

There are better explanations, and my explanation may be incorrect, although the substance is similar and sufficient to identify major differences between linear and nonlinear equations.

I suggest that the reader look at
Chaos: Making a New Science
Paperback – August 26, 2008
by James Gleick
Available on Amazon:
Audiobook 1 Credit Paperback $16.71
Available at Thriftbooks.com for 4.19

Nonlinear equations define Chaos Theory.

At a starting point there is stability.

However, nonlinear equations describe instability created by small differences or changes over time.

There are tipping points where a slight change can create a huge change. This is where the Butterfly Effect makes an impact.

Each individual in an organization has the power to create that slight change.

That small change is unpredictable in the long term. The result is that the stock market, the weather, politics, suicide, and homicide are predictable in the short term, but unpredictable in the long term.

Organizations cannot control the butterfly effect.
Organizations are unstable because all it takes is a divorce, a domestic quarrel, a stroke, a new baby, or a promotion, to change a member of the organization.

Any change can launch the Butterfly Effect.

Control is an imaginary construct and an illusion in the fog of wishful thinking.

For an introduction I suggest,
Chaos and society A. Albert (Ed.). (1995).
Chaos and society (Vol. 29). Ios Press.
The literature is large, and the reader will be overwhelmed by the amount of literature available.

Suffice it to say. All healthcare facilities are very different, even though they all rely upon the same medications, the same surgeries, the same counseling techniques, the same DSM-V etc. Slight differences in personnel create a large difference in outcomes.

The rest of this book will describe small differences in starting points that result in large differences in outcomes.

Now for the rest of the story a la Paul Harvey.

Bullying?

I am small, Chinese, and different.

I have been bullied all my life.

I never complained about it because I saw that it was pervasive and complaining seemed to do nothing but make it worse.

I do know bullying when I see it, and it is thinly veiled throughout the health care systems and society.

Minorities participate in the bullying, to the point that society is so fractured that there is no majority, and everybody is being bullied.

Most people have been bullied.

"About 6 of every 10 men (or 60%) and 5 of every 10 women (or 50%) experience at least one trauma in their lives"

PTSD: National Center for PTSD
https://www.ptsd.va.gov/understand/common/c
mmon_adults.asp

Nationwide, 81% of women and 43% of men reported experiencing some form of sexual harassment and/or assault in their lifetime. National Sexual Violence Resource Center (NSVRC) https://www.nsvrc.org/statistics "National studies of U.S. adult men and women, which found prevalence of direct physical or sexual assault victimization to be 55% among women and 66.8% among men (Tjaden & Thoennes, 1998)."

National Estimates of Exposure to Traumatic Events and PTSD Prevalence Using DSM-IV and DSM-5 Criteria
Dean G. Kilpatrick, Heidi S. Resnick, Melissa E. Milanak, Mark W. Miller, Katherine M.

Keyes, and Matthew J. Friedman
J Trauma Stress. Author manuscript; available
in PMC 2014 Oct 1.
Published in final edited form as: J
Trauma Stress. 2013 Oct; 26(5): 537–547.
doi: 10.1002/jts.21848
PMCID: PMC4096796
NIHMSID: NIHMS 596966 PMID: 24151000
https://www.ncbi.nlm.nih.gov/pmc/articles/PM4
096796/

**Bullies and Their Victims: Understanding
a Pervasive Problem in the Schools**
George M. Batsche &Howard M. Knoff Pages
165-174 | Published online: 22 Dec 2019
https://doi.org/10.1080/02796015.1994.1208574

**Bullying is pervasive in
the healthcare setting.**
"Poor staffing levels, excessive workloads,
subpar management skills, stress and lack of
autonomy are some of the factors that
contribute to bullying in the workplace—
including in medicine—according to a recent
AMA report on the problem that pervades
health care and how to stop it."

Why bullying happens in health care and how to stop it
Brendan Murphy
Senior News Writer
PHYSICIAN HEALTH
APR 2, 2021

Patients bully healthcare workers with threats, false accusations of neglect, abuse, and discrimination, and even assaults.

"Nearly 50% of emergency physicians say they've been assaulted. 70% of emergency nurses report being hit or kicked on the job. So, what's the solution?"
Rising violence in the emergency department
Ken Budd, Special to AAMC News
February 24, 2020

What is the solution to bullying? The trends towards, understaffing, exploitation and abuse of healthcare workers have survived decades of putative "solutions."
Reducing workplace bullying in healthcare organizations
Randle, Jacqueline; Stevenson, Keith; Grayling, Ian; Walker, Christine.

Nursing Standard (through 2013); London Vol. 21, Iss. 22, (Feb 7-Feb 13, 2007): 49-56; quiz 58

Every religion uses the Golden Rule, "do unto others as you would have them do unto you." This is the cure to bullying.

Unfortunately, antisocial personalities and antisocial behaviors gain traction in social organizations. With the unfair advantages of lying, stealing, cheating, intimidation, threats, and assaults the antisocial personalities have an unfair advantage in reaching the top.

"The lifetime prevalence of antisocial personality disorder (APD), conduct disorder, and adult antisocial behavior were 3.6%, 1.1%, and 12.3%, respectively. Prevalence of alcohol use disorders and drug use disorders were 30.3% and 10.3%, respectively."

Prevalence, correlates, and comorbidity of DSM-IV antisocial personality syndromes and alcohol and specific drug use disorders in the United States: results from the national epidemiologic survey on alcohol and related conditions
Wilson M Compton 1, Kevin P Conway, Frederick S Stinson, James D Colliver, Bridget

F Grant
PMID: 15960559 DOI: 10.4088/jcp.v66n0602
The prevalence of addiction and intoxication in emergency rooms increases the risks of threats, abuse, and assaults directed at health care workers.

Burnout?

There has been a growing literature on professional burnout and the retirement of many healthcare professionals which accelerated during the Covid-19 pandemic.

The issue of burnout and early retirement of healthcare professionals has been simmering for many years.

The loss of seasoned health care workers has resulted in the rise of EAP's, Employee Assistance Programs.

The employee receives evaluation, diagnosis, and treatment for a mental illness caused by the stress of working in an environment of a high patient case load, a heavy documentation burden, and short hours in which to accomplish the work.

An egregious example is nurses who were expected to work off the clock, after their eight-hour shift without pay to complete the paperwork,

Many nurses retired and then they were given higher pay and hired in greater numbers.

Creep, the tendency to add more patients with more paperwork, without additional time or pay tends to recreate the same problems over and over as MBAs, as administrators, attempt to control costs and increase profits.

This led to the EAP's (Employee Assistance Programs). Hard work was rewarded with a diagnosis of a mental illness, medication, counseling, and an Employee Appreciation Day.

When it came time for relicensure, application for malpractice insurance, review by the credentials committee for annual credentialling, the healthcare **workers were burdened with responding to inquiries**

about mental illness and fitness for work as a healthcare professional. No good deed goes unpunished?

Before Covid-19 there was literature on Burnout. There were Employee Assistance programs. The health care worker was given an evaluation, a diagnosis of mental illness and treatment of mental illness.

"46 percent of physicians," suffered burn out. "Lower patient satisfaction and care quality, Higher medical error rates and malpractice risk, Higher physician and staff turnover, Physician alcohol and drug abuse and addiction, Physician suicide.
Yes, burnout can be a fatal disorder. Suicide rates for both men and women are higher in physicians than the general population and widely underreported.9"
Physician Burnout: Its Origin, Symptoms, and Five Main Causes Burnout is everywhere, but you can't fight an enemy unless you recognize it. Dike Drummond, MD Fam Pract Manag. 2015 Sep-Oct;22(5):42-47. © 2015 Dike Drummond, MD, CEO, TheHappyMD.com

Covid-19 created a tipping point among healthcare workers.

"An overwhelming 55% of front-line health care workers reported burnout (defined as mental and physical exhaustion from chronic workplace stress)"
Medical burnout: Breaking bad
Dharam Kaushik, MD, June 4, 2021

Moral Injury?
Suddenly there was an epiphany.
Someone realized that most of the employees were stressed, but not mentally ill.

The employees were struggling with bullying and a dysfunctional work environment.

Healthcare providers are expected to take care of the sick and dying. However, the MBAs were administrators serving the stockholders first and the patients second and the employees third.
The administrative priorities were cost control, revenue stream and profits. As a result, the employees were struggling with many stakeholders in addition to the patient.

Clinicians, are forced to consider the demands of other stakeholders, the electronic medical record (EMR), the insurers, the hospital, the health care system, the peer review committee, the malpractice insurance carrier, the state licensing board, the credentialling committee, the patient, the patient's family, the community, vocal self interest groups, the judge, the jury, the prosecutor, as other players force their way into the room with the clinician and the patient.

After the meeting, all the stakeholders complete a satisfaction survey. The clinician has a peer review that includes the patient's response to treatment and the satisfaction of the patient and all the other stakeholders.

The joint commission, the hospital credentialling committee, the specialty medical boards, the electronic medical record, the risk management committee, and the peer review committee all add layers of documentation to be added during and after the visit.

Patient's, the putative primary beneficiaries, find that they spend time with clinicians who do not make eye contact, but have their faces buried into a computer screen during the "face to face," contact that is the basis for submitting billing to the insurance company?

Patient satisfaction goes down the toilet because of the documentation requirements.

Quality of care, well, the clinician is now a data entry clerk, and the administrative chain of command now can push a button and create impressive spreadsheets.

The administrators are looking real good. The cash flow is really good. Clients don't like their clinicians looking into the computers while talking to the clients.

'Death by 1000 Cuts': Medscape National Physician Burnout & Suicide Report 2021
Leslie Kane, MA | January 22, 2021

https://www.medscape.com/slideshow/2021-lifes tyle-burnout-6013456

Burnout is properly redefined as moral injury and "These routine, incessant betrayals of patient care and trust are examples of 'death by a thousand cuts.' Any one of them, delivered alone, might heal. But repeated on a daily basis, they coalesce into the moral injury of health care."
Physicians aren't 'burning out.' They're suffering from moral injury
By Simon G. Talbot and Wendy Dean
July 26, 2018
https://www.statnews.com/2018/07/26/physicians-not-burning-out-they-are-suffering-moral-injury/

The healthcare system has been suffering from pressure to provide more paperwork and more care with fewer providers for decades.

Minimalist Management strategies taught in MBA programs is the primary driving force. **Minimalist Management is** the practice of hiring the minimum **number of people, who are the least qualified, and lowest paid to**

generate a revenue stream with minimal costs.

This results in health care services having a chain of command with non-physicians at the top because physicians are expensive.

Any time you put a non-physician supervisor between the CEO and the physician provider the revenue stream creates a disconnect between the best medical practice and the patient care.

"The number of physicians in the United States grew 150 percent between 1975 and 2010, roughly in keeping with population growth, while the number of **healthcare administrators increased 3,200 percent** for the same time period."
Expert Forum: The rise (and rise) of the healthcare administrator By Joe Cantlupe | November 7, 2017, https://www.athenahealth.com/knowledge-hub/ practice-management/expert-forum-rise-and-ris e-healthcare-administrator

The Great Healthcare Bloat: 10 Administrators for Every 1 U.S. Doctor
https://www.healthline.com/health-news/policy-ten-administrators-for-every-one-us-doctor-092813

"By far the biggest culprit of the mushrooming workload is the electronic medical record, or E.M.R. It has burrowed its tentacles into every aspect of the healthcare system."

The Business of Health Care Depends on Exploiting Doctors and Nurses

One resource seems infinite and free: the professionalism of caregivers.

June 8, 2019

© 2022 The New York Times Company
https://www.nytimes.com/2019/06/08/opinion/sunday/hospitals-doctors-nurses-burnout.html

Arbitrary time limits with the patient does not allow for the best practice of medicine.

The best practice requires a complete assessment, even if the client is depressed, confused, disorganized, speaks through an interpreter and slow to answer questions.

The best practice requires informed choice.

That means that time must be taken to educate the client as to what the risks and benefits are and time for the client to make that choice.

Is the provider seeing 5, 10, 15, 20, 25, 30 "clients," a day?

At what point is the contact a fly by with the work product a billable progress note, a prescription and a mere salute to the best practice of informed choice?

Who in the chain of command sets the appointment schedule for the doctor. I doubt that it is the doctor.
The doctor wades through the list, talking to the "clients," writing a progress note and prescribing a pill and salutes "informed choice," during the fly by. How many patients are on the list before the doctor is wearing the Emperor's New Clothes and merely posturing?

Reporting Bullying and Moral Injury?
Who is tasked with reporting bullying and moral injury in the healthcare workplace?

The government has web sites,
"stopbullying.gov," is an official government
website designed to reduce bullying.

Osha addresses bullying in the workplace.
https://www.ccohs.ca/oshanswers/psychosocial/
bullying.html

What is workplace bullying?
"Bullying is usually seen as acts or verbal
comments that could psychologically or
'mentally' hurt or isolate a person in the
workplace. Sometimes, bullying can involve
negative physical contact as well. Bullying
usually involves repeated incidents or a
pattern of behavior that is intended to
intimidate, offend, degrade, or humiliate a
particular person or group of people. It has also
been described as the assertion of power
through aggression."
Health consequences of bullying in the
 healthcare workplace: A systematic review
医护服务工作场所欺凌行为会带来的健康后果:系

统性评价 Isabel Lever BA (Hons), MD, Daniel
Dyball BSc (Hons), Neil Greenberg MD, Sharon
A. M., Stevelink PhD

First published: 28 February 2019
https://doi.org/10.1111/jan.13986Citations: 28

Theoretically anyone can, and everyone should
report bullying in the workplace.

It looks good on paper, but it really doesn't
work that way in the real world.

The Failure to Protect Whistleblowers?
"Frontline workers ...do not come forward due
to the fear of retaliation they have and remain
silent."

The Failures of Whistleblower Laws in
Protecting Workers - is unionization the
remedy to ensure compliance with cyber-
security laws? By Alvin Velazquez1 Sean
Hansen2 Despite all of these efforts, frontline
workers in the financial sector and other
sectors covered by the patchwork of state and
federal whistleblower laws do not come forward
due to the fear of retaliation they have and
remain silent.

"Whistleblowers are left open to retaliation
despite new laws to protect them."

A FAILURE OF WHISTLEBLOWER
PROTECTION
BROKEN GOVERNMENT
The Center for Public Integrity
Published — December 10, 2008Updated —
May 19, 2014, at 12:19 pm ET
How America fails its whistleblowers who work
with classified information have a few options.
All of them are bad.
By Ranjani Chakraborty and Laura Bult Nov
27, 2019, 10:00am EST

**Why is it so difficult to provide informed
choice in the medical setting?**
Science has been corrupted by politics and
money.

Pharmaceutical companies do not publish all
the information necessary to provide informed
choice.

Federal regulatory agencies have been
captured by the pharmaceutical industry.

Protecting Pharmaceutical Companies and the
Revenue Streams of Pharmaceutical
Companies has a priority over patient safety in
federal regulatory agencies.

Protecting revenue streams in healthcare agencies has taken priority over patient safety.

Internal politics in healthcare agencies has taken priority over patient and staff safety.

Let me insert Old Wisdom here. Old Wisdom has stood the test of time and has survived the rise and fall of empires, churches, fads, and hysterias for millennia.

First,
"No Good Deed Goes Unpunished."
Do not expect Whistleblower laws to protect you. Do not expect integrity from your chain of command. Be prepared to deal with antisocial personalities and antisocial behaviors in every setting that you find yourself in. Accept bullying as a condition of employment anywhere. Do not expect Good Deeds to be rewarded.

Second, Murphy's Law,
"Sooner or later if it can go wrong, it will go wrong."
If you see a risk in your workplace, know that it will happen sooner or later and you will be a part of the outcome, depending upon your

behavior prior to the perfection of that risk in death or another bad outcome.

Do not expect any mercy from the plaintiff attorney.

Third, Pandora's Box.
Do not play with Pandora's Box.
Do not open Pandora's Box.
Once the evil in Pandora's box is released it cannot be put back.

Just ask any president. The most powerful person in the world cannot put it back into Pandora's Box. President Clinton famously said, "I did not have sex with that woman." President Nixon famously said, "I am not a crook."

When attorneys get a hold of information they will extract their pound of flesh,
Ford Motor company looked at Pinto safety and The Pinto Memo: 'It's Cheaper to let them Burn!' The result was $128,000,000 in punitive damages rendered by the jury.
https://www.spokesman.com/blogs/autos/2008/o ct/17/pinto-memo-its-cheaper-let-them-burn/

And
**The Completely Preventable Disaster of
The Exploding Ford Pinto**
T G Writes
Updated July 28, 2021
https://www.ranker.com/list/exploding-ford-
pinto/tracey-graham

The Crisis in Science
There has been a crisis in science for decades.
Scientific research that is published can't be
reproduced by other scientists. Unless the
research can be reproduced, it is not sound
science.

**1,500 scientists lift the lid on
reproducibility** Monya Baker nature news
feature article Published: 25 May 2016
Nature volume 533, pages452–454 (2016)
The crisis in scientific publications is getting
worse. Interesting research is more likely to be
published if it is interesting even if it is not
science that can be replicated by other
scientists.
**"Papers that cannot be replicated are
cited 153 times more because their
findings are interesting, according to a**

new UC San Diego study."
A New Replication Crisis: Research that is Less Likely to be True is Cited More
May 21, 2021, | By Christine Clark
https://ucsdnews.ucsd.edu/pressrelease/a-new-replication-crisis-research-that-is-less-likely-be-true-is-cited-more?fbclid=IwAR3Eiqlm-hdMJTZ70FnhLv8WpMg5WrGTvnvX5aIlwx75dB4Qt OQon4jlnA

If a healthcare professional does not have the correct information, how is informed choice even possible?

Misinformation provided by pharmaceutical companies.

It would seem that all businesses and multinational corporations have a tendency to promote bad science in support of their revenue streams and narratives. The welfare of the public is a secondary consideration for the purposes of window dressing and deflection.

Trial sans Error: How Pharma-Funded Research Cherry-Picks Positive Results
Clinical trial data on new drugs is systematically withheld from doctors and

patients, bringing into question many of the premises of the pharmaceutical industry—and the medicine we use
By Ben Goldacre on February 13, 2013, Published by Faber and Faber, Inc. © 2013 Ben Goldacre. Scientific American
https://www.scientificamerican.com/article/trial-sans-error-how-pharma-funded-research-cherry-picks-positive-results/

"The boundaries between academic medicine — medical schools, teaching hospitals, and their faculty — and the pharmaceutical industry have been dissolving since the 1980s, and the important differences between their missions are becoming blurred. Medical research, education, and clinical practice have suffered as a result."
Ex-editor of NEJM tells how Big Pharma has corrupted academic institutions
In the May/June issue of the Boston Review, Dr. By Susan Perry

Federal Regulatory Agencies No Longer Protect American Citizens from Pharmaceutical Companies.

The FDA used to protect the United States

Citizens from the Pharmaceutical industry.

An FDA director was decorated by President
Kennedy for saving lives and protecting United
States Citizens.
"President John F. Kennedy, in August 1962,
awarding Dr. Frances Oldham Kelsey the
President's Medal for Distinguished Federal
Civilian Service for her exceptional judgment
in evaluating the drug Thalidomide. Dr. Kelsey
was only the second woman to receive this
award—the highest honor that can be
bestowed upon a US civilian"
Commemorative Issue: Protecting the Public:
Dr. Frances Oldham Kelsey
Karen Geraghty
AMA Journal of Ethics
Illuminating the Art of Medicine
Virtual Mentor. 2001;3(11):
DOI
10.1001 /virtualmentor.2001.3.11.prol2-0111.

A lot has changed since 1972.
50 years of approval? | FDA wants over half a
century to disclose Pfizer jabs approval docs
https://www.youtube.com/watch?v=4u62p5KCF
tE
FDA Says It Now Needs 75 Years to Fully

Release Pfizer COVID-19 Vaccine Data
Coronavirus, FDA, Pfizer, Coronavirus Vaccine
Posted on All Sides December 8th, 2021
https://www.allsides.com/news/2021-12-08-
1553 /fda-says-it-now-needs-75-years-fully-
release-pfizer-covid-19-vaccine-data

Ivermectin is on the WHO (World Health
Organization) list of safe and essential
medications...ivermectin Tablet (scored): 3 mg
https://apps.who.int/iris/bitstream/handle/1066
5/325771/WHO-MVP-EMP-IAU-2019.06-
eng.pdf
"Conclusions:
Moderate-certainty evidence finds that large
reductions in COVID-19 deaths are possible
using ivermectin. Using ivermectin early in the
clinical course may reduce numbers
progressing to severe disease. The apparent
safety and low cost suggest that ivermectin is
likely to have a significant impact on the
SARS-CoV-2 pandemic globally."
**Ivermectin for Prevention and Treatment
of COVID-19 Infection: A Systematic
Review, Meta-analysis, and Trial
Sequential Analysis to Inform Clinical
Guidelines**

Bryant, Andrew MSc1, *; Lawrie, Theresa A.
MBBCh, PhD2; Dowswell, Therese PhD;
Fordham, Edmund J. PhD2; Mitchell, Scott
MBChB, MRCS3; Hill, Sarah R. PhD1; Tham,
Tony C. MD, FRCP4Author Information

American Journal of Therapeutics: July/August
2021 - Volume 28 - Issue 4 - p e434-e460
THERAPEUTIC ADVANCES
doi: 10.1097/MJT.0000000000001402
https://journals.lww.com/americantherapeutics/
fulltext/2021/08000/ivermectin_for_prevention_
and_treatment_of.7.aspx

"Ivermectin fights 21 viruses, including SARS-
CoV-2, the cause of Covid-19. A single dose
reduced the viral load of SARS-CoV-2 in cells
by 99.8% in 24 hours and 99.98% in 48 hours,
according to a June 2020 study published in
the journal Antiviral Research."
"In 115 patients with Covid-19 who received a
single dose of ivermectin, none developed
pneumonia or cardiovascular complications,
while 11.4% of those in the control group did.
Fewer ivermectin patients developed
respiratory distress (2.6% vs. 15.8%); fewer
required oxygen (9.6% vs. 45.9%); fewer
required antibiotics (15.7% vs. 60.2%); and

fewer entered intensive care (0.1% vs. 8.3%).

Ivermectin-treated patients tested negative faster, in four days instead of 15, and stayed in the hospital nine days on average instead of 15.

Ivermectin patients experienced 13.3% mortality compared with 24.5% in the control group."

"Despite the FDA's claims, ivermectin is safe at approved doses. Out of four billion doses administered since 1998, there have been only 28 cases of serious neurological adverse events, according to an article published this year in the American Journal of Therapeutics. The same study found that ivermectin has been used safely in pregnant women, children and infants."

Why Is the FDA Attacking a Safe, Effective Drug?
Ivermectin is a promising Covid treatment and prophylaxis, but the agency is denigrating it. By David R. Henderson and Charles L. Hooper July 28, 2021 12:34 pm ET

https://www.wsj.com/articles/fda-ivermectin-cov id-19-coronavirus-masks-anti-science-11627482 393

There is bad science, there is bullying in health care, the pharmaceutical industry promotes bad science, the federal regulatory agencies protect the pharmaceutical industry.

How does a clinician give informed consent to a patient in real time?

In order to give the patient informed consent, the physician must be able to tell the patient what the risks and benefits of the medication are.

The physician is often misinformed by the medical literature for a variety of reasons.

First there is publication bias. Publication bias: For a fact check and deeper look I refer the reader to:
Publication bias in meta-analyses from the Cochrane Database of Systematic Reviews
Michal Kicinski David A. Springate Evangelos Kontopantelis

First published: 18 May 2015
https://doi.org/10.1002/sim.6525

For more information I refer the reader to:
Not to be confused with Reporting bias or
Media bias. Publication bias is a type of bias
that occurs in published academic research. It
occurs when the outcome of an experiment or
research study influences the decision whether
to publish or otherwise distribute it. Publishing
only results that show a significant finding
disturbs the balance of findings and inserts
bias in favor of positive results.[1] The study of
publication bias is an important topic in
metascience. Studies with significant results
can be of the same standard as studies with a
null result with respect to quality of execution
and design.[2] However, statistically
significant results are three times more likely
to be published than papers with null
results.[3] A consequence of this is that
researchers are unduly motivated to
manipulate their practices to ensure that a
statistically significant result is reported.[4]
From Wikipedia, the free encyclopedia
I will leave it to the reader to research the
following list of flaws in research regarding the
risks and benefits of psychotropic medications.

Research fails to include pregnant women and children on ethical grounds.

Research fails to include elderly and people with multiple medical problems.

Research fails to include people on multiple medications.

Small sample size is not sufficient to provide reliable data.

Samples are not random because they do not include people who refuse.

Samples are not random because populations may not be accessible.

Studies are not randomized.

Studies are not blinded.

Studies do not use the same criteria for diagnosis or target symptoms.

The studies are of short duration.

Studies do not clearly separate spontaneous remission from medication effect.

Studies do not account for cognitive dissonance in addition to placebo effect.

It is difficult to identify altered data, "fudging."

This is not even the tip of the iceberg. One study uncovered **710 unique research flaws** for excluding research from evidence-based databases.

For fact checking and a deeper look at the shortcomings of medical research I refer the reader to:

A Large-Scale Analysis of the Reasons Given for Excluding Articles that are Retrieved by Literature Search During Systematic Review Tracy Edinger, ND, MCR and Aaron M. Cohen, MD, MS AMIA
Annu Symp Proc. 2013; 2013: 379–387.
Published online 2013 Nov 16.
PMCID: PMC3900186
PMID: 24551345

Addicting Medications, No Functional Recovery The Long View
Your Nineteenth Psychiatric Consultation
William R. Yee M.D., J.D.
Copyright Applied for January 1st, 2021

It is difficult for the physician to wade through an extensive medical literature and weed out the truth from the false research results being published.

"Considering that these surveys ask sensitive questions and have other limitations, it appears likely that this is a conservative estimate of the true prevalence of scientific misconduct."

How Many Scientists Fabricate and Falsify Research? A Systematic Review and Meta-Analysis of Survey Data

Daniele Fanelli
Published: May 29, 2009
https://doi.org/10.1371/journal.pone.0005738

Prevalence of Research Misconduct and Questionable Research Practices:

A Systematic Review and Meta-Analysis
Yu Xie, Kai Wang & Yan Kong
Practices: A Systematic Review and Meta-Analysis. Sci Eng Ethics 27, 41 (2021).
https://doi.org/10.1007/s11948-021-00314-9
August 10, 2018 @@
"Findings: In this systematic review of 265 studies comprising 400 647 drug samples and meta-analysis of 96 studies comprising 67 839 drug samples, the prevalence of substandard and falsified medicines in low- and middle-income countries was 13.6% overall (19.1% for antimalarials and 12.4% for antibiotics). Data on the estimated economic impact were limited primarily to market size and ranged widely from $10 billion to $200 billion."

Prevalence and Estimated Economic Burden of Substandard and Falsified Medicines in Low- and Middle-Income Countries A Systematic Review and Meta-analysis

Sachiko Ozawa, PhD, MHS, Daniel R. Evans, MSc; Sophia Bessias, MPH; et al Deson G. Haynie, MHS; Tatenda T. Yemeke, MSc; Sarah K. Laing, MPH2; James E. Herrington, PhD

JAMA Netw Open. 2018;1(4):e181662. doi:10.1001/jamanetworkopen.2018.1662

"Both publication bias and outcome reporting bias may affect meta-analyses, and the effect can be unpredictable. Adding unreported data from both published and unpublished drug trials to 41 meta-analyses caused 46% of the meta-analytic effect estimates to show lower efficacy of the drug, 7% to show identical efficacy, and 46% to show greater efficacy."

Preferred reporting items for systematic review and meta-analysis protocols (PRISMA-P) 2015: elaboration and explanation

Larissa Shamseer, David Moher, Mike Clarke, Davina Ghersi, Alessandro Liberati (deceased), Mark Petticrew, Paul Shekelle,

Lesley A Stewart7the PRISMA-P Group BMJ
2015; 349 doi:
https://doi.org/10.1136/bmj.g7647 (
Published 02 January 2015)
Cite this as: BMJ 2015;349:g7647

Let us examine the antipsychotic medications.

An early large-scale examination of the
effectiveness of antipsychotics was the CATIE
trials.

**Perphenazine is as effective as
olanzapine, quetiapine, risperidone, and
ziprasidone.**

Perphenazine is the most cost-effective
medication for the treatment of psychosis.

**You can expect three out of four patients
to stop antipsychotic medications** within
eighteen months due to side effects or
failure of benefit to justify the time and
money to continue the treatments.

See:

**"What CATIE Found: Results From the
Schizophrenia Trial,"** Dr. Marvin S.
Swartz, M.D., T. Scott Stroup, M.D., M.P.H.,
Dr. Joseph P. McEvoy, M.D., Dr.
Sonia M. Davis, Dr.P.H., Dr. Robert A.

Rosenheck, M.D., Dr. Richard S. E. Keefe, Ph.D., Dr. John K. Hsiao, M.D., and Dr. Jeffrey A. Lieberman, M.D.;
Psychiatr Serv.
2008 May; 59(5): 500–506.;
doi: 10.1176/ps.2008.59.5.500; PMCID: PMC5033643;   NIHMSID: NIHMS816833;
PMID: 18451005

There are many criticisms of the CATIE trials. See:

"CATIE & You, What happens when drugs are found to be unsafe and ineffective? Not much," by Ben Hansen, MindFreedom Michigan, Ragged Edge Online Home

The CATIE Schizophrenia Trial involved 1493 patients with schizophrenia treated for up to 18 months with

olanzapine ....7.5 to 30 mg per day,
perphenazine ....8 to 32 mg per day,
quetiapine ....200 to 800 mg per day,
risperidone ....1.5 to 6.0 mg per day,
Ziprasidone ....40 to 160 mg per day,

74 percent of patients discontinued their medication before 18 months

64 percent of those assigned to olanzapine,

74 percent of those assigned to perphenazine
82 percent of those assigned to quetiapine
74 percent of those assigned to risperidone
79 percent of those assigned to ziprasidone.

CONCLUSIONS
Patients discontinued medications for
intolerable side effects or lack of benefit
sufficient to justify the adverse effects and cost
in time and money.

**Effectiveness of Antipsychotic Drugs in
Patients with Chronic Schizophrenia**

Jeffrey A. Lieberman, M.D., T. Scott Stroup,
M.D., M.P.H., Joseph P. McEvoy, M.D., Marvin
S. Swartz, M.D., Robert A. Rosenheck, M.D.,
Diana O. Perkins, M.D., M.P.H., Richard S.E.
Keefe, Ph.D., Sonia M. Davis, Dr.P.H.,
Clarence E. Davis, Ph.D., Barry D.
Lebowitz,Ph.D., Joanne Severe, M.S., and John
K. Hsiao, M.D.
September 22, 2005
N Engl J Med 2005; 353:1209-1223 DOI:
10.1056/NEJMoa051688
"Adverse effects are likely to be the most
common reason for patients to not comply with
prescribed medication regimens.

Ineffectiveness, complexity of the regimen and cost are also important medication-related factors contributing to noncompliance."

Noncompliance with Medication for Psychiatric Disorders
Reasons and Remedies
Robert Breen & Joshua T. Thornhill
Disease Management
Published: 14 September 2012
CNS Drugs volume 9, pages457–471 (1998)
"For example, the results of our recent telemedicine study, showed that the compliance rate, among schizophrenic patients with symptomatic remission, in the first month of the treatment was 44.6%, and had been decreasing over the subsequent 6 months (Krzystanek et al. 2015)."

RISK FACTORS FOR NONCOMPLIANCE WITH ANTIPSYCHOTIC MEDICATION IN LONG-TERM TREATED CHRONIC SCHIZOPHRENIA PATIENTS
Marek Krzystanek, Krzysztof Krysta, Maágorzata Janas-Kozik, Ewa Martyniak & Janusz Rybakowski
Psychiatria Danubina, 2019; Vol. 31, Suppl. 3, p 543-548 Conference paper ©

The standard of care is, "Informed Choice."
The best practice is, "the lowest effective dose."
Informed Choice requires that the psychiatrist
inform the patient of the risks and benefits.
The lowest effective dose is the dose that gives
the maximum benefit with the minimum side
effect.

**The Choice remains the patient's choice
and not the doctor's choice.**
The very concept of medication noncompliance
is a violation of the standard of "Informed
Choice," as "Noncompliance," transfers the
choice from the patient to the doctor.
If the patient finds the side effects
unacceptable, then the lowest effective dose is
no medication at all.
If the family, hospital, Peer Review, or other
"stakeholder" is not satisfied with the patient's
choice we are no longer in a doctor patient
relationship.

The place of the "Stakeholders" in the equation
needs to be evaluated through the lens of
"Informed Choice," and "the lowest effective
dose."

Which stakeholder has the power to impose his or her will on the patient?
Is it the spouse, parent, child, teacher, Peer Review Committee,
State Licensing Board, Credentialling Committee, Malpractice Insurance Carrier?

I will let each reader decide for themselves.

Corporate America has a long history of lying, cheating and stealing to boost profits.

I refer the reader to the following:
In the best of all possible worlds, science should provide a guide for progress of political, business, and social evolution.
However, in the real world, politics and business corrupt science and political evolution.
The sugar industry actively redirected science, politics and social evolution away from the risks of sugar, obesity, diabetes and heart disease to red meat and fat.
For a fact check and a deeper look I refer the reader to
50 Years Ago, Sugar Industry Quietly Paid Scientists To Point Blame At Fat

September 13, 20169:59 AM ET
CAMILA DOMONOSKE
and:

**Sugar Industry and Coronary Heart
Disease Research**
**A Historical Analysis of Internal
Industry Documents**

Cristin E. Kearns, DDS, MBA1,2; Laura A.
Schmidt, PhD, MSW, MPH1,3,4; Stanton A.
Glantz, PhD1,5,6,7,8
Author Affiliations

JAMA Intern Med. 2016;176(11):1680-1685.
doi:10.1001/jamainternmed.2016.5394
November 2016

This was not a first, but a part of a long history
of big business creating fake science to support
a revenue stream.
For a fact check and deeper look I refer the
reader to the asbestos coverup:
Review:
**The Dusting of America: A Story of
Asbestos: Carnage, Cover-Up, and
Litigation**
**Reviewed Work: Outrageous Misconduct:
The Asbestos Industry on Trial**

by Paul Brodeur
Review by: David Rosenberg
Harvard Law Review
Vol. 99, No. 7 (May, 1986), pp. 1693-1706 (14 pages)
Published By: The Harvard Law Review Association

https://doi.org/10.2307/1341085
https://www.jstor.org/stable/1341085

For a fact check and deeper look into the Tobacco Industry I refer the reader to:
Smokescreen: The Truth Behind the Tobacco Industry Cover-up
Robert N. Proctor, PhD
Author Affiliations
JAMA. 1996;276(12):998.
doi:10.1001/jama.1996.03540120076040
September 25, 1996

The pharmaceutical industry has a long record of misinformation and abuse of them market place.
For a fact check and deeper look into Neurontin/gabapentin I refer the reader to:
Pfizer to Pay $420 Million in Illegal Marketing Case

By Kenneth N. Gilpin

New York Times

May 13, 2004

In regards a fact check and deeper look into illegal marketing and pleading guilty to criminal charges I refer the reader to:

"In May 2004, Pfizer agreed to pay $430 million and to plead guilty to criminal charges for illegally marketing Neurontin for unapproved uses such as migraine headaches and pain."

Pfizer to pay $325 million in Neurontin settlement

By Jonathan Stempe JUNE 2, 20149:55 AM UPDATED 7 YEARS AGO

For a fact check and deeper look into Oxycontin I refer the reader to:

OxyContin maker Purdue Pharma pleads guilty to criminal charges

HEALTHCARE & PHARMA

NOVEMBER 24, 2020; 12:10 PMU PDATED 12 mDAYS AGO   By Mike Spector

and:

OxyContin Maker To Pay Out Billions In Civil, Criminal Penalties

October 22, 2020 5:06 AM ET
LAW NPR
Heard on Morning Edition
BRIAN MAN
**Addicting Medications, No Functional
Recovery, The Long View Your
Nineteenth Psychiatric Consultation
William R. Yee M.D., J.D.
Copyright Applied for January 1st, 2021**

**In my office it is
"Informed Choice," and,
"The Lowest Effective Dose," and the
arbiter of those issues is:
the client and:
only the client .**

**Let us examine the process
of informed choice.**
The client is examined and diagnosed with
schizophrenia, schizoaffective disorder, bipolar
disorder, depression with psychotic symptoms,
or a diagnosis with hallucinations, delusions
and or paranoia appropriate for antipsychotic
medications.

The diagnosis cannot be confirmed by x-ray, blood test, or other basis that is as specific as the identification of a bacteria in pneumonia.

The diagnosis is a guess based upon a collection of symptoms, but the cause is not known.

Because we really don't know what mental illness is on the same sound basis that we know what bacterial pneumonia is, we cannot know what the mechanism of action of antipsychotic medication is.

"**The dopamine hypothesis of schizophrenia** postulates that postsynaptic dopamine antagonism is the common mechanism that explains antipsychotic properties."

The dopamine hypothesis of schizophrenia embraces the thought that first-generation (typical) antipsychotics are D2 antagonists. The dopamine hypothesis of schizophrenia embraces the thought that second-generation antipsychotics include 5-HT2A antagonism, fast D2 dissociation, and 5-HT1A agonism.

Mechanism of Action of Antipsychotic Agents
Flavio Guzman, M.D. Psychopharmacology
Institute
https://psychopharmacologyinstitute.com/publi
cation/mechanism-of-action-of-antipsychotic-
agents-2094

"**The mechanism of action** of most first-
and second-generation antipsychotics (FGAs
and SGAs) **appears to be** postsynaptic
blockade of brain dopamine D2 receptors."
**Second-generation antipsychotic
medications: Pharmacology,
administration, and side effects**
Author: Michael D Jibson, MD, PhD. Section
Editor: Stephen Marder, MD Deputy
Editor: Michael Friedman, MD

The Number Needed to Treat? NNT?
You offer the client a choice of medications and
advise the patient that:
 Discontinuation rates for antipsychotics are
.....olanzapine 64%
.....risperidone ...74%
.....perphenazine 75%
.....ziprasidone ...79%

From the patient's perspective the
psychiatrist must treat
3 patients with olanzapine
for 1 patient to get better
4 patients with risperidone
for 1 patient to get better
4 patients with perphenazine
for 1 patient to get better
5 patients with ziprasidone
for 1 patient to get better
sufficiently for the patient to be willing to
continue the medication.

**The CATIE Schizophrenia Trial: Results,
Impact, Controversy**

Theo C. Manschreck , MD, MPH &Roger A.
Boshes , MD, PhD

Pages 245-258 | Received 16 Mar 2007,
Accepted 15 Jun 2007, Published online:
03 Jul 2009

Then you introduce the patient to the concept
of NNH, the Number Needed to Harm.
Doctors lack information about how often
patients suffer side effects. For this reason
doctors lack the ability to give complete
information for informed choice. Doctors cannot
tell patients how many patients are treated

with a medication for one patient to suffer harm. NNH is the number of patients treated for one patient to suffer harm.

It has been known for decades that medication side effects, including death, are underreported.

For 60 years, underreporting has plagued the FDA system for tracking drug side effects

John Fauber, Milwaukee Journal Sentinel
https://www.jsonline.com/story/news/investigations/2020/11/30/underreporting-has-plagued-fda-side-effects-tracking-system/6339395002/

Haloperidol therapy with dementia may be associated with 1 additional death for every 26 patients receiving treatment. NNH is 26 with death being the harm.

Haloperidol had the highest risk of death and quetiapine had the least risk of death.

Risperidone and olanzapine increased the death rate more than quetiapine.

Finally higher doses of antipsychotics have higher death rates.

Quetiapine increased mortality by 2.0%, yielding an NNH of 50

Quetiapine has the least mortality, but less benefit than olanzapine or risperidone.

Antipsychotics, Other Psychotropics, and the Risk of Death in Patients With Dementia Number Needed to Harm
Donovan T. Maust, MD, MS; Hyungjin Myra Kim, ScD; Lisa S. Seyfried, MD, MS; et al Claire Chiang, PhD; Janet Kavanagh, MS; Lon S. Schneider, MD, MS; Helen C. Kales, MD
Author Affiliations Article Information
JAMA Psychiatry. 2015;72(5):438-445. doi:10.1001/jamapsychiatry.2014.3018

There is a Block Box Warning in the FDA labels for antipsychotic medications because it is known that antipsychotics cause death in elderly patients with dementia.

What about the elderly without dementia? Are antipsychotic medications safe with the elderly without dementia?

"Conclusions
Prevalence of potentially inappropriate
medications in nursing homes according to the
NORGEP-NH was extensive, and especially
the use of multiple psychotropic drugs. The
high prevalence found in this study shows that
there is a need for higher awareness of
medication use and side effects in the elderly
population."

**Potentially inappropriate medication use
in nursing homes: an observational study
using the NORGEP-NH criteria**

Gunhild Nyborg, Mette Brekke, Jørund
Straand, Svein Gjelstad, and Maria Romøren

BMC Geriatr. 2017; 17: 220.
Published online 2017 Sep 19. doi:
10.1186/s12877-017-0608-z
PMCID: PMC5606129
PMID: 28927372

"Conclusions
This study found that psychiatric patients in
contact with a CMHS have an almost twofold
higher mortality rate than the general
population. These findings demonstrate that,
since the closure of long-stay psychiatric
hospitals, the physical health care of people
with mental health problems is often neglected

and clearly requires greater attention by health-care policymakers, services and professionals."

Mortality and cause of death among psychiatric patients: a 20-year case-register study in an area with a community-based system of care
L. Grigoletti, G. Perini, A. Rossi, A. Biggeri, C. Barbui, M. Tansella and F. Amaddeo
Published online by Cambridge University Press: 20 April 2009

"The FDA black box warning that use of atypical antipsychotic medications in elderly patients with dementia nearly doubled the risk of death, clinicians, patients and caregivers are left with unclear choices for treating people with dementia with psychosis and/or severe agitation."

Antipsychotic treatments for the elderly: efficacy and safety of aripiprazole Izchak Kohen, Paula E Lester, and Sum Lam
Neuropsychiatr Dis Treat. 2010; 6: 47–58.
Published online 2010 Mar 24. doi: 10.2147/ndt.s6411
PMCID: PMC2846120
PMID: 20361061

Elderly patients with schizophrenia are a particularly vulnerable group often excluded from clinical trials.
Currently there is no evidence-synthesis about the efficacy and safety of antipsychotics in this subgroup."

Antipsychotic drugs for elderly patients with schizophrenia: A systematic review and meta-analysis

Marc Krause 1, Maximilian Huhn , Johannes Schneider-Thoma , Philipp Rothe , Robert C Smith 3, Stefan Leucht
Affiliations expand

Meta-Analysis Eur Neuropsychopharmacol. 2018 Dec;28(12):1360-1370. doi: 10.1016/j.euroneuro.2018.09.007.
Epub 2018 Sep 20.
PMID: 30243680 DOI: 10.1016/j.euroneuro.2018.09.007

"There is no trial-based evidence upon which to base guidelines for the treatment of late-onset schizophrenia."

Antipsychotic drug treatment for elderly people with late-onset schizophrenia

Adib Essali 1, Ghassan Ali

Review Cochrane Database Syst Rev.

2012 Feb 15; 2012(2):CD004162.
doi:10.1002/14651858.CD004162.pub2.
PMID: 22336800 PMCID: PMC6986693
DOI: 10.1002/14651858.CD004162.pub2

The bottom line is that there is no basis for concluding that antipsychotic medication is safer to use in the elderly without dementia than elderly patients with dementia.

The elderly, in general, have declining physiologic reserves and tolerate adverse medication effects less than the young and healthy. That is why the elderly are more likely to die with the flu or a pandemic.

Another measure of the benefit is what percentage of symptoms are removed in response to the medication.

The range is zero percent, 0%, to one hundred percent, 100%.

Zero would be no benefit and one hundred percent would be a cure.

For psychotropic medications 20% reduction of symptoms is sufficient for the FDA to give approval for marketing the medication for the treatment of mental illness.

A 40% reduction of symptoms is a "robust," response from the point of view of the pharmaceutical industry.

The pharmaceutical industry is interested in a revenue stream and there is a great temptation to lie, steal and cheat based upon the fines and criminal prosecutions listed above.

From the viewpoint of the patient, family and significant others a cure is desired. Twenty to forty percent reduction of symptoms is not a cure and fifty to seventy five percent of patients stop taking psychotropic medications after eighteen months.

Is that fifty to seventy five percent who stop taking antipsychotic medications properly classified as noncompliance or a vote of no confidence?

Clozaril-Clozapine

Let us examine Clozaril, a putative "Gold Standard," in the treatment of severe mental illness, especially Schizophrenia.

Clozaril is prescribed when mentally ill patients fail to respond to other antipsychotic medications.

Let us examine some of the available literature on Clozaril.

Keep in mind there is a replication crisis in science, there is publication bias, bad research is more likely to be cited and found than good research, pharmaceutical companies often publish misleading research or present and most importantly, side effects are under reported as cited above.

Results

A total of 108 studies revealed an incidence of clozapine-associated

neutropenia..3.8%

severe neutropenia...................................0.9%

Death was......................................0.013%

Fatality of severe neutropenia was..2.1%

The prevalence of agranulocytosis and related death in clozapine-treated patients: a comprehensive meta-analysis of observational studies

Published online by Cambridge University Press: 12 March 2019

Xiao-Hong Li,, Xiao-Mei Zhong,, Li Lu, Wei Zheng,, Shi-bin Wang,, Wen-wang Rao

Background

Clozapine treatment increases the risk of agranulocytosis, but the epidemiology of agranulocytosis has been inconsistent.

Results

Studies with 260,948 clozapine-treated patients published between 1984 and 2018 reveal:

prevalence of agranulocytosis 0.4%
death caused by agranulocytosis........... ..0.05%

The prevalence of agranulocytosis and related death in clozapine-treated patients: a comprehensive meta-analysis of observational studies

Xiao-Hong Li, Xiao-Mei Zhong, Li Lu, Wei Zheng, Shi-Bin Wang, Wen-Wang Rao, Shuai Wang, Chee H Ng, Gabor S Ungvari, Gang

Wang, Yu-Tao Xiang
Meta-Analysis Psychol Med. 2020
Mar;50(4):583-594. doi:
10.1017/S0033291719000369.
Epub 2019 Mar 12.
PMID: 30857568 DOI:
10.1017/S0033291719000369

Clozapine treated patients who suffered
sudden death were about 10 years younger and
healthier than non-Clozapine treated patients
who experienced sudden death. **The sudden
death rate was 3.8 times higher for
Clozapine treated patients** than for non
clozapine treated patients, whereas the rate of
disease-related death was 5 times higher for
non-clozapine treated patients than for
clozapine treated patients.
**The rate of suicide among patients
currently receiving clozapine in this
sample was 3.6 times higher than among
non-clozapine treated patients.**
Because clozapine treated patients who
experienced sudden death were also younger
and healthier, it seems that **treatment with**

clozapine may present a greater risk for sudden death than treatment with other psychiatric medications.

Sudden death in patients receiving clozapine treatment: a preliminary investigation

I Modai, S Hirschmann, A Rava, R Kurs, P Barak, P Lichtenberg, M Ritsner Case Reports J Clin Psychopharmacol. 2000 Jun;20(3):325-7.
PMID: 10831019
DOI: 10.1097/00004714-200006000-00006

Mortality rate ratios were not significantly lower in patients ever treated with clozapine during follow-up, but significantly lower in patients continuously treated with clozapine compared to patients with other antipsychotics

Potentially fatal outcomes associated with clozapine

Kevin J. Liabc, Ronald J. Gurreraabc, Lynn E. Delisiabc

Schizophrenia Research
Volume 199, September 2018, Pages 386-389

Abstract
Morbidity and mortality associated with

clozapine includes risk of agranulocytosis, aspiration pneumonia, bowel ischemia, myocarditis, seizures, and weight gain. Mortality with clozapine induced myocarditis can be 24%.

Long term all-cause mortality can be 22%. About 43% were diagnosed with diabetes compared to a national prevalence of 13.7%. Clozapine can cause death by cardiovascular and other medical disorders.

Clozapine, Diabetes Mellitus, Cardiovascular Risk and Mortality: Results of a 21-Year Naturalistic Study in Patients with Schizophrenia and Schizoaffective Disorder

Katlyn L Nemani, M Claire Greene, Melissa Ulloa, Brenda Vincenzi, Paul M Copeland, Sulaiman Al-Khadari, David C Henderson
PMID: 29164928 PMCID: PMC6489443 DOI: 10.3371/CSRP.KNMG.111717

There is not a scientific basis to determine which antipsychotic is more effective for patients with treatment-resistant schizophrenia. Blinded Random Controlled Trials in contrast to unblinded, randomized effectiveness studies do not provide evidence of the superiority of clozapine compared with other second-generation antipsychotics"

Efficacy, Acceptability, and Tolerability of Antipsychotics in Treatment-Resistant Schizophrenia: A Network Meta-analysis
Myrto T Samara, Markus Dold, Myrsini ianatsi, Adriani Nikolakopoulou, Bartosz Helfer, Georgia Salanti, Stefan Leucht Meta-Analysis JAMA Psychiatry. 2016 Mar;73(3):199-210. doi: 10.1001/jamapsychiatry.2015.2955. PMID: 26842482 DOI: 10.1001/jamapsychiatry.2015.2955

Clinicians must monitor WBC and granulocyte counts and may wish to consider weekly hematologic monitoring for the duration of clozapine therapy. Abrupt agranulocytosis may occur at any time.

Sudden Late Onset of Clozapine-Induced Agranulocytosis
Nick C Patel, Peter G Dorson, Tawny L Bettinger
First Published June 1, 2002 Case Report Find in PubMed https://doi.org/10.1345/aph.1A417

"There are two major classes of ADRs: (1) unpredictable, uncommon and idiosyncratic, and (2) predictable, common and dose-related [4]. The latter are better described as related to serum concentrations [5]. There is recent agreement among the most important medical scientists, such as Vanderbroucke and Psaty [6] or Ioannidis [7], that the status of ADR science is highly deficient. According to them, there are two main reasons for the poor status of ADR knowledge [6, 7]: (1) pharmaceutical companies tend to try to minimize the existence of ADRs, and (2) rare but potentially lethal ADRs, usually idiosyncratic, are usually not detected by the randomized clinical trials (RCTs) required for drug approval, since they are short-term and include only a few thousand patients. These deficiencies have led to several drugs being withdrawn from the market due to unidentified potentially lethal ADRs [8]."

A Rational Use of Clozapine Based on Adverse Drug Reactions, Pharmacokinetics, and Clinical Pharmacopsychology

de Leon J., Ruan C.J.d, Schoretsanitis G., De las Cuevas C.

Psychother Psychosom 2020;89:200–214
https://doi.org/10.1159/000507638

Clozapine-Clozaril through the lens of the FDA Label

The FDA Label is the most convenient and comprehensive source of information available to the practicing clinician for the evaluation and use of medications.

The FDA Label for most medications will list hundreds of effects and side effects including:
Black Box warnings for death in demented geriatric paitients.
Birth Defects
Myocarditis
Leukopenia
Neuroleptic Malignant Syndrome
Constipation
Tardive Dyskinesia
Toxic Symptoms of Overdose
Withdrawal Syndromes-Rebound Symptoms
Literally hundreds of side effects

Let us examine the FDA Label for Clozaril as a tool for giving the patient informed choice.

This is done knowing that side effects are under reported and pharmaceutical companies have a history of exaggerating benefits and minimizing side effects in research data.

I leave it to the reader to determine how much the benefits are exaggerated and how much the adverse effects are minimized.

I have not found the perfect method for sorting these matters out, after fifty years as a practicing physician, with diligence in monitoring the literature and educating patients about medications.

I start by telling the patient that they should report all new physical symptoms as any symptom can be a medication side effect, previously known, or waiting to be discovered.

Second, I tell my patients that with psychiatric medications, the safest thing to do if a side effect emerges is to stop the medications, go to an emergency room for serious side effects and or make an appointment to adjust medications for minor side effects.

The client is stuck with determining what a serious, life-threatening side effect is.

I suggest rash, itching, difficulty breathing, difficulty maintaining consciousness and rational thinking are likely to be emergencies.

I suggest that the client read the package insert for a list of side effects or look the for FDA label online.

If the client is in my office, I will give the client a copy of the FDA Label and review it with them.
The FDA Label for Clozaril reports:
BOXED WARNING
1. AGRANULOCYTOSIS
2. SEIZURES
3. MYOCARDITIS
4. OTHER ADVERSE CARDIOVASCULAR
 AND RESPIRATORY EFFECTS
5. INCREASED MORTALITY IN ELDERLY
 PATIENTS WITH DEMENTIA-
    RELATED PSYCHOSIS
I will advise the patient that there is no sound basis for believing that Clozaril/Clozapine is safer in elderly patients without dementia.

I will advise the patient that physiologic reserves decline with age and with chronic medical conditions such as obesity, diabetes, high blood pressure and other medical abnormalities.

Additional Risks include:
1. Hyperglycemia and Diabetes Mellitus
2. Neuroleptic Malignant Syndrome (NMS)
3. Neuroleptic Malignant Syndrome (NMS)
4. Fever
5. Pulmonary Embolism
6. Hepatitis
7. Anticholinergic Toxicity
8. fecal impaction and paralytic
9. anticholinergic effects aggravating prostatic enlargement
10. Interference with Cognitive and Motor Performance
11. Cerebrovascular adverse events
Pregnancy Category B
The effects on pregnancy are not adequately studied and unknown and the medication should be avoided as much as possible during pregnancy.

OVERDOSAGE

Human Experience The most commonly reported signs and symptoms associated with CLOZARIL® (clozapine) overdose are: altered states of consciousness, including drowsiness, delirium and coma; tachycardia; hypotension; respiratory depression or failure; hypersalivation.

Aspiration pneumonia and cardiac arrhythmias have also been reported. Seizures have occurred in a minority of reported cases.

Fatal overdoses have been reported with **CLOZARIL, at doses above 2500 mg**. There have also been reports of patients **recovering from overdoses well in excess of 4 g.**

After the client is educated as to the risks of Clozapine, the client is educated as to benefits of Clozapine.

According to the Clozapine FDA Label The effectiveness of CLOZARIL in a treatment-resistant schizophrenic population was demonstrated in a

6-week study comparing CLOZARIL and chlorpromazine.

Patients meeting DSM-III criteria for schizophrenia and having a mean BPRS total score of 61 were demonstrated to be treatment resistant by history and by open, prospective treatment with haloperidol before entering into the double-blind phase of the study.

The superiority of CLOZARIL to chlorpromazine was documented in statistical analyses employing both categorical and continuous measures of treatment effect "Patients who met the multiple psychiatric symptom criteria were then randomly assigned to a **six-week double-blind treatment trial with either clozapine (up to 900 mg/d) or chlorpromazine and benztropine mesylate (up to 1800 mg/d of chlorpromazine hydrochloride and up to 6 mg of Benztropine mesylate).**" "Average daily doses of active antipsychotic medication received during double-blind treatment are shown by treatment week in Fig 1. Adequate dose levels of each drug were attained with mean peak dosages exceeding 1200 mg/d of chlorpromazine and 600 mg/d of clozapine. The decrease in average dosage for both treatment groups at week 6 reflects the mandated taper-down at the end of the treatment period for all patients, designed to avoid abrupt discontinuation."

BPRS total score C

Clozapine ....126 Patients

Baseline Score   61 ±12

Endpoint Score 45 ± 13

Chlorpromazine ....139 Patients

Baseline Score   61 ±11

Endpoint Score 56 ± 12

Two-Tailed Analysis of Covariance, P < .001

BPRS cluster of four key items

Clozapine ....126 Patients

Baseline Score 19 ± 04

Endpoint Score 14 ± 05

Chlorpromazine 139 Patients

Baseline Score 19 ± 04

Endpoint Score 17 ± 04

Two-Tailed Analysis of Covariance, P < .001

The criteria for defining a patient as improved reduction

greater than 20% from baseline in the BPRS total score

plus

a posttreatment CGI Scale score of 3 (mild) or less

or

a posttreatment BPRS total score of 35 or lower

It was found that only
4% of patients treated with chlorpromazine and benztropine had improved, while 30% of clozapine-treated patients had improved.

Clozapine for the treatment-resistant schizophrenic. A double-blind comparison with chlorpromazine

J Kane 1, G Honigfeld, J Singer, H Meltzer
Clinical Trial Arch Gen Psychiatry 1988 Sep;45(9):789-96. doi: 10.1001/archpsyc.1988.01800330013001. PMID: 3046553 DOI: 10.1001/archpsyc.1988.01800330013001

My first comment is that there is a large subjective element involved in the BPRS. A total of 265 severely mentally ill patients were found with an average baseline score of 61 with a plus minus of 11 or 12.

A total of 265 patients were found with a score of 19 plus minus 4 on four key indicators. First you must know what a BPRS Score is. BPRS is short for Brief Psychiatric Rating Scale

The rater is asked to render his opinion on 18 aspects of mental illness.

From a range of zero to seven, least to worst he will give his opinion on the severity of each aspect of mental illness in the BPRS That means the range of scores is from 0 to 126.

My second comment is that based upon this I should inform my patients that if they want to accept a therapeutic trial of Clozapine, they can expect a 30% chance of a 20% improvement.

The client can expect 3 out of ten patients to benefit from clozapine. That is about 1 out of 3 patients will benefit by taking Clozaril.

I suppose if the client thought the mental illness was very severe, the client might be willing to accept death as an alternative to mental illness.

The adverse effects of Clozaril include severe physical illness and death. The risk is so high that the patient must accept weekly blood tests to continue taking the Clozaril.

Because of the severity of adverse effects, treatment of patients failing to show a clinically significant response should not continue

What is a clinically significant response? Ask the patient.

The need for continuing treatment in patients with clinical responses should be periodically reevaluated.

The client should be offered a medication taper as an option with each visit to determine the continued need for clozapine. It is always the patient's choice based upon the patient's willingness to accept risks for benefits.

Thank you for your time and attention.
I am here to do no harm, and help if I can.

William R. Yee M.D., J.D.
Board Certified Psychiatrist.
Practicing Medicine and Psychiatry without interruption since 1972 in Michigan, Indiana, Kentucky, California and Texas

"Pre-Existing text," includes names of symptoms and medical illnesses, medications, people, corporations, law cases, statutes, text of statutes, the titles of articles and books, the content of FDA Labels, articles and books cited.

My copyright claim is a clam to the "original text," which is my personal experiences as described in the text above and my commentary on the names of symptoms and medical illnesses, medications, people, corporations, law cases, statutes, text of statutes, the titles of articles and books, the content of FDA Labels, articles and books cited.